GUT HEALTH UNLOCKED

The Mindful Path to Quick Digestion Relief, Lasting Weight Loss and Easy Leaky Gut Repair

DENISE SMITH MARSH

© Copyright Denise Smith Marsh 2024 - All rights reserved.

The content within this book may not be reproduced, duplicated or transmitted without direct written permission from the author or the publisher.

Under no circumstances will any blame or legal responsibility be held against the publisher, or author, for any damages, reparation, or monetary loss due to the information contained within this book. Either directly or indirectly. You are responsible for your own choices, actions, and results.

Legal Notice:

This book is copyright protected. This book is only for personal use. You cannot amend, distribute, sell, use, quote or paraphrase any part, of the content within this book, without the consent of the author or publisher.

Disclaimer Notice:

Please note the information contained within this document is for educational and entertainment purposes only. All effort has been expended to present accurate, up-to-date, and reliable, complete information. No warranties of any kind are declared or implied. Readers acknowledge that the author is not engaging in the rendering of legal, financial, medical or professional advice. The content within this book has been derived from various sources. Please consult a licensed professional before attempting any techniques outlined in this book.

By reading this document, the reader agrees that under no circumstances is the author responsible for any losses, direct or indirect, which are incurred as a result of the use of the information contained within this document, including, but not limited to, — errors, omissions, or inaccuracies.

CONTENTS

Introduction — 7

1. YOUR GUT IN A NUTSHELL — 11
   1.1 The Gut-Brain Connection: Unlocking the Mood-Digestion Link — 11
   1.2 Microbiome 101: Your Gut's Ecosystem and Its Inhabitants — 13
   1.3 From Acid to Enzymes: The Digestive Process Demystified — 15
   1.4 Leaky Gut Syndrome: The What, Why, and How — 18
   1.5 SIBO and Its Impact: Understanding Small Intestinal Bacterial Overgrowth — 22

2. NAVIGATING THE GUT HEALTH MAZE: MYTHS AND REALITIES — 27
   2.1 Understanding Probiotics — 27
   2.2 Gluten-Free: Necessity or Trend? — 30
   2.3 Detox Diets: Helpful or Harmful? — 33
   2.4 Dairy Dilemmas: Intolerance vs. Sensitivity — 37
   2.5 The Low-FODMAP Diet: Not a One-Size-Fits-All Solution — 40

3. TAILORING YOUR DIET FOR GUT HEALTH — 43
   3.1 Identifying Your Gut's Needs: A Self-Assessment Guide — 43
   3.2 Anti-Inflammatory Foods: Your Gut's Best Friends — 46
   3.3 Prebiotics and Probiotics: Balancing Your Gut Flora — 49
   3.4 The Importance of Fiber: Types, Sources, and Benefits — 53
   3.5 Integrating Fermented Foods: A Practical Approach — 56

4. SPECIAL DIETS AND THEIR ROLE IN GUT HEALTH — 59

- 4.1 The Gluten-Free Lifestyle: Beyond Celiac Disease — 59
- 4.2 The Low-FODMAP Journey: Navigating Digestive Relief — 61
- 4.3 The Ketogenic Diet: Impacts on the Gut Microbiome — 65
- 4.4 Vegan and Vegetarian Diets: Pros and Cons for Gut Health — 68
- 4.5 Elimination Diets: Finding What Works for You — 71

5. UNRAVELING THE STRESS-GUT CONNECTION — 75

- 5.1 The Vicious Cycle: Stress, Cortisol, and Your Gut — 75
- 5.2 Meditation and Mindfulness: Tools for Stress Reduction — 77
- 5.3 Sleep's Role in Gut Health: Connecting the Dots — 81
- 5.4 Exercise and Gut Health: Finding the Right Balance — 84
- 5.5 Time Management: Reducing Stress for Better Digestive Health — 87

6. NOURISHING THE FOUNDATION - HYDRATION AND ROUTINE FOR OPTIMAL GUT HEALTH — 95

- 6.1 The Role of Hydration: Water's Impact on Digestion — 95
- 6.2 Herbal Remedies and Supplements: What Works? — 98
- 6.3 The Power of Routine: Structuring Your Day for Gut Health — 101
- 6.4 Healing the Gut-Brain Axis: A Mindful Approach — 105
- 6.5 Environmental Factors: Your Surroundings and Your Gut — 107
- 6.6 Intermittent Fasting and Gut Health — 110
- 6.7 Detoxification and Gut Health — 113

7. UNRAVELING COMMON GUT CHALLENGES — 117

- 7.1 Navigating Persistent Bloating: Causes and Solutions — 117
- 7.2 Combating Chronic Constipation: A New Approach — 121

7.3 Dealing with Diarrhea: Dietary and Lifestyle Changes	124
7.4 Tackling Food Intolerances Head-On	127
7.5 Overcoming the Anxiety of Eating Out with Gut Issues	130
8. GUT HEALTH AND WEIGHT MANAGEMENT	133
8.1 The Microbiome-Weight Connection	134
8.2 Dietary Strategies for a Balanced Microbiome	136
8.3 Mindfulness and Weight Loss	139
9. DEMYSTIFYING THE GUT HEALTH CONUNDRUMS	143
9.1 Do Probiotics Work for Everyone? Understanding the Variability	143
9.2 Can Gut Health Affect My Mood and Energy Levels?	145
9.3 Is It Too Late to Improve My Gut Health?	148
9.4 How Can I Tell If My Gut Health Is Improving?	151
9.5 Combating Skepticism: Why Natural Remedies Deserve a Place in Your Gut Health Toolkit	155
10. CRAFTING YOUR PATH TO GUT HEALTH	159
10.1 Setting Realistic Goals for Gut Health Improvement	159
10.2 Tracking Your Progress: Tools and Techniques	161
10.3 Adjusting Your Plan: When to Pivot and Why	166
10.4 Community Support: Finding Your Gut Health Tribe	169
10.5 Staying Motivated: Celebrating Wins and Overcoming Setbacks	172
Conclusion	177
References	181

INTRODUCTION

Several years ago, on a morning that began like any other, I found myself doubled over in pain, the kind that commands your full attention. This pain wasn't a new sensation, but a profound realization struck me on this day: our gut health forms the basis of our overall well-being. That moment marked the beginning of a transformative journey for me and the countless individuals I've had the privilege to help since co-founding a weight loss and wellness clinic seven years ago. This journey, rich with discovery, challenges, and triumphs, is the foundation of "Gut Health Unlocked: The Mindful Path to Quick Digestion Relief, Lasting Weight Loss, and Easy Leaky Gut Repair."

This book is more than just a guide; it's a mission to offer a holistic approach to improving gut health, specifically designed for adults over 40. After years of seeing clients struggle with conventional methods, I realized a dire need for a comprehensive, accessible, personalized plan. Our goal is to address this need, providing you with a pathway to understand, effectively manage, and improve your gut health.

My hands-on experience in the wellness clinic, coupled with rigorous research and collaboration with health experts, has equipped me with unique insights into the challenges and solutions related to gut health. This book distills those years of experience and learning into an accessible guide aimed at those who feel they've tried it all to no avail.

You, the reader, are at the heart of this book. If you're over 40 and seeking a sustainable, evidence-based approach to gut health that considers your unique needs and lifestyle, you've found your guide. With a blend of personal anecdotes, scientific explanations, practical advice, and real-life success stories, "Gut Health Unlocked" offers a comprehensive exploration of achieving optimal gut health.

We'll delve into the latest research on the gut-brain axis, illuminating how our digestive health is inextricably linked to our mental and physical wellness. This book is structured to walk you through the essentials of gut health, from understanding its foundational importance to implementing dietary and lifestyle changes that have proven effective for many. Each chapter builds on the next, creating a clear, actionable plan tailored to your needs.

What sets this book apart is its commitment to providing personalized, evidence-based strategies. We recognize that there is no one-size-fits-all solution to gut health. By incorporating real success stories, we aim to inspire and motivate you to embark on your journey confidently, armed with the knowledge that change is possible.

As you turn these pages, I encourage you to reflect on your gut health journey and what you hope to achieve. To enhance your experience, consider journaling your observations, challenges, and successes as you apply the insights and strategies discussed.

By the end of this book, you'll have a deeper understanding of your gut health and a personalized plan to improve it. This is my promise to you. Let's start this journey together with open minds and the shared goal of unlocking the full potential of our gut health for a happier, healthier life.

YOUR GUT IN A NUTSHELL

The moment you step into a bustling kitchen, the rich aroma of cooking envelops you, signaling your stomach to prepare for the impending feast. This visceral, almost instantaneous response showcases the intricate dance between our bodies and brains - a dance led by an often overlooked organ: the gut. This chapter will delve into the complex connection between the gut and the brain. This connection significantly impacts our mood, cognitive abilities, and overall wellness.

1.1 THE GUT-BRAIN CONNECTION: UNLOCKING THE MOOD-DIGESTION LINK

At the heart of this connection is the vagus nerve, a veritable highway of communication that runs directly from the brain to the gut. It transmits signals in both directions, allowing for a continuous exchange of information. This bi-directional communication network is known as the gut-brain axis. Through this pathway, our digestive system doesn't just process food; it also sends and receives crucial signals that affect our emotional and mental states.

One of the most fascinating aspects of this communication is the role of neurotransmitters, chemicals responsible for transmitting messages throughout the body. Serotonin, often dubbed the 'feel-good' neurotransmitter due to its mood-regulating properties, is predominantly produced in the gut, not the brain, as commonly assumed. This revelation underscores the gut's potential influence over our psychological well-being. When the gut microbiome— the vast ecosystem of microorganisms living in our digestive tract —is balanced, serotonin production is optimized, promoting a sense of calm and happiness. However, when this delicate balance is disrupted, whether by poor diet, stress, or antibiotics, it can lead to a decrease in serotonin, contributing to feelings of depression and anxiety.

The stress response further illustrates the gut-brain axis's impact on our health. In stressful situations, the brain signals the gut, often leading to gastrointestinal symptoms such as butterflies in the stomach or, in more severe cases, nausea. This response is the body's immediate reaction to stress, mediated by the gut-brain connection. On the other hand, a disrupted digestive system can send signals to the brain, causing increased levels of stress or anxiety, which in turn can create a vicious cycle that is difficult to break. This highlights the importance of maintaining gut health not only for digestive wellness but also for mental health.

Given these intricate connections, adopting a holistic approach to health is crucial. This approach promotes gut health through a balanced diet, exercise, stress management, and sleep. These practices support a healthy gut microbiome, promoting optimal neurotransmitter production and a balanced stress response. For example, incorporating fermented foods like yogurt and kimchi into one's diet can boost the gut's production of beneficial bacteria. At the same time, mindfulness and meditation practices can modulate the stress signals sent along the vagus nerve, reducing the impact of stress on the gut.

Integrating these strategies can significantly improve digestive and mental health, underscoring the power of the gut-brain connection. Acknowledging and addressing this connection can unlock new pathways to health and well-being, demonstrating that a happy gut contributes to a happy mind.

1.2 MICROBIOME 101: YOUR GUT'S ECOSYSTEM AND ITS INHABITANTS

Imagine your gut as a bustling metropolis, where trillions of microorganisms coexist in a delicate balance, including bacteria, viruses, fungi, and protozoa. This vast, dynamic community is known as the gut microbiome, and it plays a pivotal role in your health, from aiding digestion to bolstering your immune system. These microscopic inhabitants are the unsung heroes of your well-being, working tirelessly behind the scenes to keep your body functioning optimally.

The significance of the microbiome extends beyond digestion. It's intricately involved in protecting against pathogens, synthesizing essential vitamins, and even regulating inflammation. A well-balanced microbiome is akin to a well-tuned orchestra, with each microorganism playing its part in harmony. Disruption of this balance can result in various health issues, such as inflammatory bowel diseases, mental health disorders, and obesity. This underscores why fostering a diverse microbiome is crucial for maintaining good health.

A kaleidoscope of factors influences the diversity of your gut's ecosystem. Diet, for instance, is a significant player. Fiber-rich foods, such as fruits, vegetables, and whole grains, support the growth and activity of beneficial bacteria. On the other hand, a diet high in processed foods and sugars can feed harmful bacteria, tipping the scales towards imbalance. Lifestyle choices, including physical activity and sleep patterns, also significantly impact the microbiome. Regular exercise increases microbial diversity, while lack of sleep can disrupt the gut's microbial balance. Environmental exposures, including antibiotics and pollutants, can further alter the microbiome, often with long-lasting effects.

Nurturing your microbiome, therefore, involves a holistic approach that encompasses diet, lifestyle, and mindful intervention when necessary. Incorporating various plant-based foods can enhance microbial diversity, introducing beneficial bacteria and feeding those already present. Fermented foods, rich in natural probiotics, such as yogurt, kefir, and sauerkraut, offer another avenue to bolster your gut's inhabitants. Prebiotic foods, including onions, garlic, and asparagus, provide the fuel to help these beneficial bacteria thrive.

In addition to dietary changes, incorporating probiotic supplements can offer a targeted approach to improving microbiome health, especially after disruptions such as antibiotic treatment. However, wisely choosing these supplements is essential, focusing on strains and quantities that address specific health needs or concerns.

Regular physical activity is a crucial lifestyle aspect supporting a healthy microbiome. Consistent exercise contributes to overall health and positively impacts the diversity and composition of the gut microbiome. This relationship demonstrates how our bodily systems are interconnected and underscores the significance of a holistic approach to health.

Finally, reducing exposure to antibiotics and environmental pollutants can help preserve the delicate balance of your gut's ecosystem. While antibiotics are sometimes necessary, their indiscriminate use can decimate the beneficial bacteria in the gut, leading to imbalances. Mindfulness and advocating for reasonable use can protect your microbiome from unnecessary harm.

By embracing these strategies, you can support and enhance the health of your gut microbiome, paving the way for improved digestion, immunity, and overall well-being.

1.3 FROM ACID TO ENZYMES: THE DIGESTIVE PROCESS DEMYSTIFIED

Digestion is a complex, finely-tuned process that begins when food touches your lips and ends when waste leaves your body. Central to this process are stomach acid and digestive enzymes, critical players in breaking down food into nutrients your body can absorb and use.

Digestion Overview

Once you start eating, your body springs into action. Saliva, rich in enzymes, begins the breakdown of carbohydrates. As you swallow, the food travels down the esophagus and reaches the stomach, where it encounters stomach acid. This acidic environment serves multiple purposes: it starts breaking down proteins, acts as a disinfectant by killing off potential pathogens in food, and creates the right conditions for enzymes to work effectively. From there, the semi-digested food moves to the small intestine, where most nutrient absorption occurs. Here, bile from the liver and many digestive enzymes from the pancreas and intestinal lining break down fats, proteins, and carbohydrates into their most minor components for absorption.

Enzyme Production

Digestive enzymes are produced in various locations throughout the digestive system, including the saliva glands, stomach, pancreas, and small intestine. Each type of enzyme has a specific role: amylases break down carbohydrates, proteases handle protein, and lipases are responsible for fat digestion. The pancreas is particularly crucial in this process, releasing enzymes into the small intestine, where they continue the digestive work started in the stomach.

Common Digestive Issues

Many common digestive complaints can be traced to imbalances or deficiencies in stomach acid and enzymes. Conditions such as heartburn, bloating, gas, and irregular bowel movements often indicate that the digestive process is not functioning as smoothly as it should. For instance, low stomach acid can lead to improper protein digestion, creating a breeding ground for bacteria and resulting in bloating and gas. Similarly, insufficient enzyme production can mean that foods aren't fully broken down, leading to nutrient malabsorption and discomfort.

Improving Digestive Health

Healthy digestion involves a blend of dietary, supplementary, and lifestyle adjustments. Here are some strategies:

- Mindful Eating: Slow down and chew your food thoroughly. Chewing mechanically breaks down food and signals the body to begin the digestive process, starting with enzyme release in the saliva.
- Balance Your Meals: Incorporate a balance of carbohydrates, proteins, and fats in your meals. This ensures a varied intake of nutrients and aids in the optimal release and functioning of different digestive enzymes.
- Stay Hydrated Adequate water intake is crucial for digestion. It helps break down food, allows for smooth passage through the digestive tract, and facilitates nutrient absorption.
- Manage Stress: High stress levels can negatively affect your digestive system, leading to reduced energy production and an imbalance in stomach acid. Deep breathing, yoga, and mindfulness can help manage stress levels.
- Supplement Wisely: In some cases, supplementing with digestive enzymes or betaine HCL (for stomach acid) can be beneficial, especially if you're experiencing signs of enzyme deficiency or low stomach acid. However, consulting with a healthcare professional before starting any supplementation is essential.

- Incorporate Fermented Foods: Fermented foods naturally contain beneficial bacteria and digestive enzymes. Including foods like yogurt, kefir, sauerkraut, and kombucha in your diet can support digestive health.
- Limit Processed Foods: Processed foods often contain additives that can disrupt the digestive process and decrease enzyme activity. Focusing on whole, unprocessed foods can help maintain a healthy digestive system.
- Regular Exercise: Physical activity is known to stimulate digestion and can help maintain regular bowel movements.

By incorporating these strategies, you can support your digestive system in performing its essential functions, improving nutrient absorption and overall health. Remember, the digestive process is a cornerstone of well-being, and taking steps to ensure its optimal function can benefit your health.

1.4 LEAKY GUT SYNDROME: THE WHAT, WHY, AND HOW

Leaky gut syndrome, though not a term you'll often hear in conventional medical circles, plays a crucial role in the health dialogue among nutritionists, holistic health practitioners, and those delving into the depths of how the gut influences overall wellness. At its core, leaky gut syndrome refers to increased intestinal permeability, where the small intestine's lining becomes damaged, allowing undigested food particles, toxic waste products, and bacteria to "leak" through the intestines and flood the bloodstream. This condition is often linked with various health issues, from digestive problems to autoimmune diseases.

Defining Leaky Gut

The intestinal lining is a barrier controlling what gets absorbed into the bloodstream. An intact and functioning barrier is selective, only allowing nutrients to enter while keeping harmful substances out. However, when this barrier becomes permeable, substances that typically wouldn't enter the bloodstream pass through, leading to an immune response. Symptoms of leaky gut can be as broad and varied as digestive disturbances, chronic fatigue, skin issues like eczema, and food sensitivities, with the condition also being associated with more severe health problems like inflammatory bowel diseases, autoimmune diseases, and even mood disorders.

Causes of Leaky Gut

The exact cause of leaky gut is still a matter of research and debate. Still, several factors have been identified as potential culprits:

- Diet: A diet high in processed foods, sugar, and certain harmful fats can contribute to the breakdown of the intestinal barrier.
- Stress: Chronic stress impacts gut health significantly, leading to changes in gut permeability.
- Antibiotics and Medications: Overusing antibiotics, non-steroidal anti-inflammatory drugs (NSAIDs), and other medications can damage the gut lining.
- Toxins: Exposure to toxins, including alcohol and environmental pollutants, can also compromise the intestinal barrier.

- Infections: Certain bacterial infections can trigger or exacerbate leaky gut syndrome.

Impact on Health

When the gut becomes permeable, it sets the stage for systemic inflammation and can trigger an immune response. For some, this might manifest as a food allergy or sensitivity, as the immune system reacts to food particles that have entered the bloodstream. Over time, this chronic inflammatory state can lead to more severe conditions, including autoimmune diseases where the body's immune system mistakenly attacks its tissues. The connection between a leaky gut and autoimmune conditions lies in the immune system's response to the constant influx of foreign particles into the bloodstream, potentially leading to an autoimmune cascade.

Repairing the Gut

Addressing leaky gut involves a multifaceted approach, focusing on diet, lifestyle, and sometimes supplementation to support healing and restore the integrity of the gut lining.

- Dietary Changes: The first step in healing a leaky gut is often adjusting one's diet. Eliminating foods that irritate the gut or trigger an immune response is crucial. This typically includes processed foods, refined sugars, and, for some individuals, gluten and dairy. Incorporating anti-inflammatory foods that promote healing is equally important. These might consist of bone broth, known for its gut-healing properties due to its high collagen content,

and fermented foods, which introduce beneficial bacteria to aid digestion and repair.
- Gut-Healing Supplements: Certain supplements can support the healing process. L-glutamine, an amino acid, is vital in repairing the intestinal lining. Omega-3 fatty acids in fish oil have potent anti-inflammatory properties that can help reduce gut inflammation. Probiotics and prebiotics are also beneficial, helping restore a healthy gut-balanced balance.
- Stress Reduction Techniques: Since stress is a significant factor in a leaky gut, finding effective ways to manage stress is essential. Practices such as yoga, meditation, and deep breathing exercises can help reduce the stress response and its impact on the gut. Regular physical activity is a powerful stress reliever and contributes to overall gut health.
- Limiting Toxin Exposure: Limiting exposure to toxins, including alcohol, NSAIDs, and environmental pollutants, can help prevent further damage to the gut lining. Becoming mindful of the products and foods one consumes can play a significant role in reducing toxin exposure.
- Restoring Sleep Patterns: Adequate sleep is crucial for gut health. Ensuring a regular sleep schedule and adopting practices that promote restful sleep can support the body's healing processes.

Taking a comprehensive approach to healing a leaky gut involves patience and persistence. Supporting the gut's natural healing processes requires sustainable changes, not quick fixes. Focusing on diet, supplementing wisely, managing stress, and being mindful of toxin exposure makes it possible to repair the gut lining, reduce inflammation, and restore balance, paving the way for improved health and well-being.

1.5 SIBO AND ITS IMPACT: UNDERSTANDING SMALL INTESTINAL BACTERIAL OVERGROWTH

Small Intestinal Bacterial Overgrowth, or SIBO, occurs when bacteria accumulate excessively in the small intestine. This condition can lead to numerous digestive discomforts, including bloating, gas, diarrhea, and abdominal pain. For adults over 40, the risk of developing SIBO increases due to factors like slower metabolism, changes in gut motility, and decreased stomach acid production, which can affect the body's ability to regulate gut bacteria effectively.

Explaining SIBO

The small intestine, typically housing a low level of bacteria, contrasts with the densely populated colon. However, when bacteria from the large intestine migrate upstream or when the small intestine's bacteria proliferate uncontrollably, SIBO can take hold. Not only does this imbalance disrupt digestion and nutrient absorption, but it also triggers inflammation and damage to the gut lining akin to the effects of leaky gut syndrome. SIBO is often challenging to diagnose and manage due to its symptoms mimicking those of other digestive disorders, requiring targeted investigation.

Causes and Risks

Several factors contribute to the development of SIBO, with impaired gut motility at the forefront. When the muscular movements of the small intestine slow down, it prevents the regular clearing of bacteria, allowing them to overgrow. Conditions such as diabetes and scleroderma can affect gut motility, as can the natural aging process. Anatomical abnormalities from surgeries or diseases that alter the small intestine's structure can also trap bacteria and foster overgrowth. Moreover, certain medications, including proton pump inhibitors, which reduce stomach acid, can create an environment conducive to bacterial overgrowth by diminishing one of the body's natural defense mechanisms against bacterial proliferation.

Diagnosis and Treatment

Diagnosing SIBO typically involves a breath test, which measures the levels of hydrogen and methane gases produced by bacteria in the mall intestine after consuming a sugar solution. Elevated levels of these gases indicate bacterial overgrowth. Treatment strategies aim to reduce bacterial overgrowth, relieve symptoms, and address the underlying causes to prevent recurrence. Antibiotics are commonly prescribed to decrease bacterial levels, with rifaximin being a popular choice due to its limited absorption and focus on the gut. In addition to medication, pro-kinetics may improve gut motility and prevent future overgrowth.

For some, a more holistic approach incorporating herbal antibiotics, such as oregano oil and berberine, has proven effective. These alternatives may offer a solution for those seeking to avoid the potential side effects of traditional antibiotics or those for whom antibiotics have not succeeded. However, it's crucial to approach these treatments under the guidance of a healthcare professional experienced in managing SIBO.

Dietary Management

The management of SIBO also heavily relies on dietary adjustments to reduce symptoms and support the gut's healing. The low-FODMAP diet, which restricts foods known to ferment in the gut and produce gas, is often recommended. This diet limits the intake of certain fruits, vegetables, grains, and dairy products known to exacerbate symptoms. While effective for many, the low-FODMAP diet is meant to be temporary, with foods gradually reintroduced to identify individual triggers and maintain nutritional balance.

In addition to the low-FODMAP diet, other nutritional strategies may include:

- Eating smaller, more frequent meals can help alleviate the burden on the digestive system, allowing it to process food more effectively and reduce bacterial fermentation.
- Limiting sugar and alcohol intake: Both can feed harmful bacteria and exacerbate SIBO symptoms.
- Incorporating gut-healing foods: Foods rich in omega-3 fatty acids, medium-chain triglycerides (like coconut oil), and bone broth can support gut healing and reduce inflammation.

Given the complexity of SIBO and its potential to mimic other digestive disorders, a nuanced approach to diagnosis and management is essential. The most efficient way to reduce symptoms and facilitate recovery from small intestine bacterial overgrowth (SIBO) is through personalized medical treatment, dietary modifications, and lifestyle changes. This highlights the significance of collaborating closely with healthcare professionals to devise a comprehensive plan that tackles the underlying causes of SIBO, alleviates symptoms, and fosters long-term gut health.

NAVIGATING THE GUT HEALTH MAZE: MYTHS AND REALITIES

Imagine walking into a supermarket, the shelves brimming with products labeled "probiotic," "gut-friendly," and "digestive health booster." It's like standing at the entrance of a labyrinth, each turn promising a shortcut to gut health nirvana. But as with any maze, there are dead ends, misleading signs, and the occasional gem waiting to be discovered. In this chapter, we'll arm you with a map to navigate this maze, starting with one of the most talked-about topics in gut health: probiotics.

2.1 UNDERSTANDING PROBIOTICS

Probiotics are live microorganisms, often called "good" or "friendly" bacteria, that confer a health benefit on the host when administered in adequate amounts. These beneficial bacteria are vital in maintaining gut health and function and are found in various foods and dietary supplements. They support the body's ability to absorb nutrients, combat harmful bacteria, and influence mood and immune function.

However, not all probiotics are created equal. Different strains have different roles, and what works for one person might not work for another. It's akin to hiring for a job; you want to match the probiotic's "skills" (its health benefits) with the "job" (your health needs).

Evaluating Probiotic Sources

There are two main avenues for probiotics: food-based probiotics and supplements.

- Food-Based Probiotics: These are naturally found in fermented foods such as yogurt, kefir, sauerkraut, kimchi, and kombucha. They're a delicious way to introduce a variety of probiotic strains into your diet. These foods often come with their own set of nutrients, offering a double whammy of health benefits. However, the quantity and quality of probiotics can vary greatly depending on factors like fermentation process and storage.
- Supplements: These offer a more targeted approach, with specific strains and dosages listed on the package. They can be beneficial for addressing particular health issues or replenishing gut flora after antibiotic use. The downside? The market is flooded with options; not all supplements are the same quality. Plus, they lack the nutritional diversity found in whole foods.

Common Misconceptions

Let's clear the air on some of the most pervasive myths about probiotics:

- More CFUs Mean Better Results: CFUs, or colony-forming units, measure the amount of live and active microorganisms in a probiotic. While it might seem logical that more CFUs would offer more significant benefits, this is only sometimes the case. Effectiveness depends on the specific strain and its role in gut health, not just the quantity.
- All Probiotics Are the Same: This couldn't be further from the truth. Different strains of probiotics serve other purposes. For example, while one strain might help digestion, another could boost the immune system more effectively.
- Immediate Results Are Guaranteed: Like planting a garden, incorporating probiotics into your regimen requires patience. It can take weeks, sometimes months, to notice changes as your gut flora gradually adjusts.

Personalized Probiotic Needs

Finding the right probiotic is a personal journey. Here are some tips for selecting a probiotic that fits your needs:

- Identify Your Health Goals: Are you looking to improve digestion, enhance immune function, or support mental health? Pinpointing your goals can help narrow down which strains might be most beneficial.

- Quality Over Quantity: Look for reputable brands that undergo third-party testing to ensure potency and purity. Don't be swayed by high CFU counts alone.
- Consider Your Diet: If you're consuming a variety of fermented foods, you might need a different approach to supplementation than someone with a limited intake of these foods.
- Consult a Healthcare Provider: It's wise to consult a healthcare professional before adding a probiotic supplement to your routine, especially if you have a health condition or are taking medication.

Navigating the world of probiotics can feel overwhelming, but armed with the proper knowledge, you can make informed choices that support your gut health journey. Remember, what works for someone else might not work for you, and that's okay. The key is to listen to your body, be patient, and adjust your approach as needed. As you explore the diverse landscape of probiotics, remember that these microorganisms are just one piece of the larger gut health puzzle. A balanced diet, regular exercise, and stress management are equally important in maintaining a healthy gut.

2.2 GLUTEN-FREE: NECESSITY OR TREND?

Recently, "gluten-free" has evolved from a medical necessity to a lifestyle choice, gracing menus and supermarket shelves alike. This surge in popularity brings to light essential distinctions between celiac disease, non-celiac gluten sensitivity, and wheat allergies, each a unique condition with its own set of challenges and needs.

Gluten Sensitivity vs. Celiac Disease

- Celiac Disease is an autoimmune disorder in which ingesting gluten damages the small intestine. It's not just about discomfort; it's about preventing harm. For those diagnosed, a gluten-free diet is not optional; it's essential for health and well-being.
- Non-Celiac Gluten Sensitivity: Here, individuals experience symptoms similar to celiac disease, including bloating, headache, or fatigue, but without the autoimmune intestinal damage. It's a gray area, often diagnosed by ruling out celiac disease and wheat allergy.
- Wheat Allergy: This involves an allergic reaction to wheat proteins, distinct from gluten. Symptoms can range from mild (rash, digestive discomfort) to severe (anaphylaxis). Avoiding wheat is crucial, but unlike celiac disease, it may not require a strictly gluten-free diet.

The Gluten-Free Diet

Adopting a gluten-free diet involves more than cutting out bread and pasta. It's a comprehensive shift that affects everything from your grocery list to social dining. While it's life-changing for those with celiac disease or gluten sensitivity, its benefits for others remain a topic of debate.

- Benefits: For those affected by gluten, removing it can lead to significant improvements in health and quality of life, including alleviation of digestive symptoms, increased energy levels, and reduced inflammation.
- Pitfalls: Jumping on the gluten-free bandwagon without medical reasons can lead to dietary imbalances. Many

gluten-free products are high in sugars and fats to compensate for texture and flavor, potentially leading to weight gain and nutritional deficiencies.

Nutritional Considerations

A well-balanced diet is critical, especially when eliminating whole categories of food, like those containing gluten. Mindful planning is required to meet nutritional needs.

- Whole Foods: Emphasize naturally gluten-free whole foods like fruits, vegetables, lean meats, fish, beans, and legumes. These provide a rich array of nutrients without the need for processed substitutes.
- Processed Gluten-Free Foods: Caution is advised as these often contain less fiber and more sugar or fat than their gluten-containing counterparts. Reading labels becomes even more important to maintain a balanced diet.
- Supplementation: Depending on individual dietary restrictions and choices, supplementing with vitamins and minerals like iron, calcium, and B vitamins might be necessary to avoid deficiencies.

Who Really Needs It?

Embarking on a gluten-free diet should not be a decision taken lightly or as a trend. It requires careful consideration and, ideally, guidance from healthcare professionals.

- Diagnosis First: Before cutting out gluten, it is crucial to get tested for celiac disease. Removing gluten prematurely can interfere with testing accuracy and lead to misdiagnosis.
- Evaluating Symptoms: A food diary tracking symptoms can be insightful for those suspecting non-celiac gluten sensitivity. Collaboration with a healthcare provider can help determine if a gluten-free diet trial is warranted.
- Beyond Digestive Health: For some, going gluten-free may stem from inflammatory or autoimmune conditions. Recent research hints at the broader impacts of gluten beyond the gut, warranting further exploration and discussion with a healthcare provider.

In navigating the choice of whether to go gluten-free, it becomes clear that personal health considerations should lead the way. For those with celiac disease or non-celiac gluten sensitivity, it's a path to relief and health. For others, it's a reminder that diet trends should be consistent with the importance of a balanced, nutrient-rich diet tailored to individual health needs and goals.

2.3 DETOX DIETS: HELPFUL OR HARMFUL?

In an era where the allure of a quick fix to flush out toxins and rejuvenate the body is stronger than ever, detox diets have surged in popularity. These diets claim to cleanse your body of toxins, improve your health, and promote weight loss by restricting certain foods and sometimes requiring specific supplements or cleansing products. The premise is appealing: reset your system by eliminating the bad and, in theory, emerge revitalized. But what does the science say, and are these diets genuinely beneficial, or could they be causing more harm than good?

Defining Detox

Detox diets typically involve a period of fasting followed by a strict diet of fruits, vegetables, fruit juices, and water. Sometimes, herbs, supplements, and teas are recommended to enhance the detox process. The underlying theory is that our bodies constantly accumulate toxins from our environment, food, and lifestyle choices, which can lead to health issues. Proponents believe that following a detox diet can rid your body of these toxins, improve your health, and even boost your energy levels.

Scientific Evidence

When you sift through the scientific literature, the support for detox diets begins to wane. The body is naturally equipped with a sophisticated detoxification system comprising the liver, kidneys, digestive system, skin, and lungs, all working together to eliminate toxins. There is little evidence to suggest that detox diets enhance this process. In fact, a review published in the Journal of Human Nutrition and Dietetics points out that there is minimal clinical evidence to support the efficacy of these diets in removing toxins from the body. Furthermore, the weight loss often associated with detox diets is typically due to fluid loss and decreased calorie intake, not the elimination of toxins. This weight is frequently quickly regained once normal eating resumes.

Potential Risks

While the promise of a quick health fix is enticing, detox diets are not without their downsides. Some potential risks are associated with these diets:

- Nutrient Deficiencies: Many detox diets are deficient in calories and may not provide all the nutrients your body needs to function optimally. Long-term adherence to such restrictive eating patterns can lead to nutrient deficiencies.
- Metabolic Disruption: Sudden and severe calorie restriction can disrupt your metabolism. Your body might respond to this perceived starvation by slowing down the metabolic rate to conserve energy, making it harder to lose weight in the future.
- Digestive Issues: Although some detox diets focus on fruits and vegetables, the lack of solid food and reliance on juices can lead to digestive discomfort, including bloating and constipation, due to low fiber intake.
- Over-reliance on Supplements: Some detox diets recommend the use of laxatives, diuretics, and other supplements to aid in cleansing. These can cause dehydration, mineral imbalances, and digestive tract issues.

Natural Detoxification Processes

Understanding that the body is already an efficient detox machine leads to a more sustainable approach to supporting its natural processes. Here's how you can aid your body's detoxification system through diet and lifestyle, without resorting to extreme detox protocols:

- Stay Hydrated: Water is crucial to the body's natural detoxification process. It helps the kidneys filter toxins and waste while retaining essential nutrients and electrolytes.

- Eat a Balanced Diet: Consuming a diet rich in fruits, vegetables, lean proteins, and whole grains ensures your body gets a wide range of nutrients, including antioxidants and fiber, which support natural detoxification processes.
- Limit Alcohol: Reducing alcohol consumption can significantly benefit liver function, one of your primary detoxification organs.
- Exercise Regularly: Physical activity encourages circulation in the blood and lymph system, enhancing detoxification. Exercise also helps you sweat, another natural way the body eliminates toxins.
- Get Enough Sleep: Adequate sleep allows your brain to reorganize and recharge itself as well as remove toxic waste byproducts that have accumulated throughout the day.
- Manage Stress: High-stress levels can negatively impact your body's detoxification ability. Stress-reduction techniques like meditation, yoga, or deep breathing exercises can support your body's natural detoxification processes.

In the quest for improved health and vitality, it's tempting to grasp the promise of a quick detox. However, understanding the body's inherent ability to cleanse itself and supporting this process through healthy lifestyle choices offers a more rational and sustainable path to wellness. Rather than seeking an external "detox" solution, focusing on nourishing your body, fostering its natural detoxification systems, and embracing a balanced approach to eating and living can lead to lasting health benefits without the risks associated with restrictive detox diets.

2.4 DAIRY DILEMMAS: INTOLERANCE VS. SENSITIVITY

Navigating the waters of dairy consumption can sometimes feel like steering through a storm without a compass. With terms like lactose intolerance and dairy sensitivity often used interchangeably, it's no wonder there's a sea of confusion. Yet, understanding these conditions is the first step to managing your diet effectively and ensuring your gut health isn't compromised.

Lactose Intolerance Explained

Lactose intolerance stems from the body's inability to digest lactose, a sugar in milk and dairy products. This intolerance occurs due to a deficiency in lactase, the enzyme responsible for breaking down lactose in the digestive system. When lactose goes undigested, it ferments in the colon, leading to bloating, gas, diarrhea, and abdominal pain. Unlike a dairy allergy, an immune response to the proteins in milk, lactose intolerance is a digestive issue that doesn't involve the immune system.

Testing for Dairy Issues

To shed light on whether discomfort after dairy consumption is due to lactose intolerance or dairy sensitivity, several tests can be quite illuminating:

- Hydrogen Breath Test: This test measures the amount of hydrogen in your breath after consuming a lactose-loaded drink. Excessive hydrogen indicates that lactose isn't being properly digested and absorbed.

- Lactose Tolerance Test: This blood test examines how well your body can digest lactose by measuring blood sugar levels before and after consuming a lactose-rich drink. A lack of significant change in blood sugar levels suggests lactose intolerance.
- Elimination Diet: Temporarily removing dairy from your diet and monitoring symptoms can be an effective approach. If symptoms improve, reintroducing dairy products one at a time can help identify specific triggers.

Alternatives to Dairy

For those looking to reduce or eliminate dairy from their diet, a variety of alternatives ensure you don't have to sacrifice taste or nutrition:

- Milk Alternatives: Almond, soy, oat, and coconut milk are popular non-dairy options, each bringing its unique flavor profile and nutritional benefits. When choosing, opt for unsweetened versions to avoid added sugars.
- Cheese and Yogurt Alternatives: Non-dairy cheese and yogurt have come a long way in taste and texture. Made from nuts, soy, or coconut, these alternatives can satisfy cravings without the discomfort dairy might cause.
- Calcium-Fortified Foods: To ensure adequate calcium intake, look for fortified non-dairy milk, juices, and cereals. Leafy greens, broccoli, almonds, and tofu are also excellent natural sources of calcium.
- Cooking and Baking: In recipes, dairy milk can often be directly substituted with a non-dairy alternative in a 1:1 ratio. For butter, coconut oil or margarine can be used,

while silken tofu or mashed bananas offer dairy-free moisture to baked goods.

Reintroducing Dairy

If you've determined through elimination or testing that you can tolerate some dairy or wish to test your tolerance, reintroducing dairy should be approached with care:

- Start Small: Begin with low-lactose foods such as hard cheeses and yogurt, which many people find easier to digest than milk.
- Gradual Increase: Slowly increase the amount and variety of dairy consumed, closely monitoring your body's response. Keeping a food diary during this period can be helpful in tracking symptoms and progress.
- Consider Lactase Supplements: For those with lactose intolerance, lactase enzyme supplements taken before consuming dairy can aid digestion and reduce symptoms.
- Listen to Your Body: Everyone's tolerance to dairy is unique. Pay attention to how your body reacts and adjust your diet accordingly. If dairy continues to cause discomfort, it may be best to limit or avoid it altogether.

Navigating dairy consumption with lactose intolerance or sensitivity doesn't have to mean missing out on delicious foods or essential nutrients. With a clear understanding of your body's responses, a wealth of dairy alternatives, and strategic dietary planning, you can enjoy a rich and varied diet that supports your gut health and overall well-being. Whether you incorporate some dairy back into your diet or opt for alternatives, the key is to listen to your body and make choices that feel right for you.

2.5 THE LOW-FODMAP DIET: NOT A ONE-SIZE-FITS-ALL SOLUTION

Imagine walking into a room filled with different keys, each promising to unlock the door to digestive comfort. Among these keys, the low-FODMAP diet has emerged as a significant tool for many grappling with digestive disorders. However, understanding its intricacies and nuances is essential before deciding if it's the correct key for you.

What Are FODMAPs?

FODMAPs are a group of carbohydrates found in certain foods that are poorly absorbed in the small intestine. The acronym stands for Fermentable Oligosaccharides, Disaccharides, Monosaccharides, And Polyols. These can draw excess fluid into the gut and undergo fermentation by bacteria in the large intestine, leading to gas, bloating, and discomfort. This is particularly relevant for individuals with Irritable Bowel Syndrome (IBS), where the gut is more sensitive to the effects of FODMAPs.

Implementing a Low-FODMAP Diet

Initiating a low-FODMAP diet requires a phased approach, traditionally starting with the elimination phase. Here, high-FODMAP foods are removed from the diet for a period—often 4 to 6 weeks—to gauge whether symptoms improve. This phase is not about long-term restriction but identifying triggers. Following this, the reintroduction phase begins, where high-FODMAP foods are gradually added back to determine personal tolerance levels. This step-by-step process helps to pinpoint specific foods that exacerbate symptoms, allowing for a more tailored, less restrictive diet moving forward.

Common Misconceptions

A prevalent misunderstanding about the Low-FODMAP diet is the perception of it as a permanent dietary overhaul. Recognizing this diet as a temporary learning tool, not a lifelong commitment, is critical. To ensure a varied and nutritionally adequate diet, the aim is to reintroduce as many high-FODMAP foods as possible, without triggering symptoms. Another misconception is that a Low-FODMAP diet benefits everyone with digestive issues. In reality, its effectiveness is most pronounced in individuals with IBS or similar functional gastrointestinal disorders.

Personalization Is Key

The cornerstone of a successful Low-FODMAP diet lies in its personalization. Here are a few strategies to tailor the diet to fit your needs:

- Work with a Dietitian: Navigating the Low-FODMAP diet can be complex. A dietitian specialized in this area can provide invaluable guidance, helping you understand which foods to avoid and how to ensure nutritional balance.
- Listen to Your Body: Pay close attention to how your body responds during each diet phase. This insight is crucial for adjusting the diet to suit your unique digestive system and lifestyle.
- Integrate Mindful Eating: Being mindful of your body's cues during meals can help identify triggers and promote a more harmonious relationship with food.

- Maintain Dietary Variety: While it's easy to focus on what's off-limits, concentrating on the variety of foods you can eat encourages a more positive and sustainable approach. This not only supports gut health but overall well-being.

The path to digestive health is as unique as the individuals walking it. The Low-FODMAP diet, focusing on personalization and discovery, offers a structured yet flexible approach to understanding one's dietary triggers. It's a tool, not a cure, designed to empower those with digestive distress to navigate their dietary choices more confidently.

As we wrap up this exploration of the Low-FODMAP diet, it's clear that the journey to gut health is multifaceted, requiring patience, experimentation, and a commitment to listening to one's body. Armed with the knowledge of FODMAPs and a personalized approach to diet, individuals can unlock the door to improved digestive health. This, coupled with a holistic view of well-being that encompasses stress management, physical activity, and adequate sleep, paves the way toward a happier gut and a more vibrant life. As we move forward, the exploration continues, delving deeper into the complex, dynamic world of gut health, where every discovery brings us closer to understanding the intricate dance of digestion and well-being.

TAILORING YOUR DIET FOR GUT HEALTH

Stepping into the realm of gut health is akin to entering a grand library, each book on the shelves representing different diets, remedies, and advice promising to soothe your digestive woes. But the true magic happens when you discover the manual written just for you, hidden among the vast collection. This chapter is your guide to creating that personalized manual, a tool to navigate the complexities of gut health with intuition, knowledge, and a pinch of wisdom.

3.1 IDENTIFYING YOUR GUT'S NEEDS: A SELF-ASSESSMENT GUIDE

Recognizing Symptoms

First things first, let's talk about tuning into your body's signals. Symptoms such as bloating, gas, irregular bowel movements, or unexplained fatigue are your body's way of sending an SOS. Ignoring these signals can lead to more significant issues down the line. Think of your body as a car; just as a dashboard light indicates something needs attention, these symptoms are clues that your digestive system may need some fine-tuning.

- Bloating: Do you feel like you've swallowed a balloon after meals? Certain foods might be causing your gut distress.
- Gas: While it's a natural part of digestion, excessive gas can be uncomfortable and a sign that not everything is in harmony in your gut.
- Irregular Bowel Movements: Too slow or too fast, neither is ideal. Your bowel habits can tell you a lot about your gut health.
- Fatigue: Ever feel like you need a nap after eating? It could be your diet rather than just a busy schedule.

Food Diary Approach

Grab a notebook or your favorite app and start tracking what you eat, how you feel afterward, and any symptoms you experience. This simple act of observation can uncover patterns you might not have noticed before. It could be that morning latte or the Friday night pizza causing trouble. Here's how to get started:

1. Date and Time: Note when you're eating as well as what you're eating.
2. Food and Drink: Write down everything, including snacks and drinks.
3. Symptoms: Record any physical reactions or feelings post-meal.
4. Emotions: Yes, how you feel emotionally can impact your gut too!

After a couple of weeks, review your diary. You might see connections between certain foods and your symptoms.

Elimination Strategy

If your food diary points to suspects causing your digestive drama, it's time to consider an elimination diet. This isn't about wholesale diet changes but rather removing one or two potential culprits for a few weeks and monitoring how you feel. Here's a step-by-step:

1. Choose Your Target: Based on your diary, select foods that are causing issues.
2. Plan Your Meals: Ensure you're still getting a balanced diet, even without these foods.
3. Monitor Closely: Keep track of any changes in symptoms or how you feel overall.
4. Reintroduction: Slowly reintroduce these foods one at a time, noting any changes.

This systematic approach can help pinpoint specific foods that don't agree with your gut. Remember, this is a tool for better understanding your body, not a restrictive diet to follow long-term.

Professional Guidance

While self-assessment and elimination diets can be illuminating, there's no substitute for professional advice. A dietitian or nutritionist can offer tailored guidance based on your symptoms, health history, and dietary needs. They can help you navigate the elimination diet more effectively, ensuring you're not missing out on essential nutrients, and can provide alternatives to keep your meals exciting and nutritious.

- **When to Seek Help:** If you're feeling overwhelmed, if symptoms persist despite your efforts, or if you have underlying health conditions, it's time to consult a professional.
- **Finding the Right Fit:** Look for a dietitian or nutritionist who has experience with gut health and can provide a personalized approach.
- **Preparation:** Before your appointment, gather your food diary, symptom tracker, and any questions. This will help you make the most of your time together.

Understanding your unique needs is the key to unlocking well-being in the vast library of gut health. By recognizing symptoms, employing a food diary, exploring elimination diets, and seeking professional guidance, you're on your way to creating a diet that supports your gut and overall health. Remember, the goal is not to find a quick fix but to develop a deeper understanding and connection with your body, leading to lasting changes that benefit your digestive system and beyond.

3.2 ANTI-INFLAMMATORY FOODS: YOUR GUT'S BEST FRIENDS

In the world of gut health, anti-inflammatory foods are akin to loyal allies, standing by to defend and nurture your digestive system. Rich in nutrients, these foods work tirelessly to calm inflammation, a root cause of many gut-related discomforts and diseases. Embracing these foods means providing your body with the tools to maintain a balanced and healthy gut environment.

Defining Anti-Inflammatory Foods

Imagine foods that taste good and possess the power to heal and protect your gut. That's the essence of anti-inflammatory foods. They are packed with vitamins, minerals, antioxidants, and omega-3 fatty acids, all of which play a pivotal role in reducing inflammation throughout the body, including the digestive tract. By incorporating these foods into your diet, you're fortifying your gut against potential invaders and soothing any irritation.

Omega-3 Rich Foods

Omega-3 fatty acids are renowned for their anti-inflammatory properties. Foods abundant in omega-3s, such as fatty fish (salmon, mackerel, and sardines) and flaxseeds, are invaluable in a gut-friendly diet. These essential fats help reduce the production of molecules and substances linked to inflammation, thereby protecting the gut lining. Including omega-3-rich foods in your meals, a few times a week can significantly reduce gut inflammation and promote overall health.

- For those not fond of fish, incorporating flaxseed into smoothies or yogurt is an excellent alternative to reap the benefits of omega-3s.

Colorful Fruits and Vegetables

The vibrant colors in fruits and vegetables aren't just for show; they signify the presence of phytonutrients, natural compounds with potent anti-inflammatory abilities. These phytonutrients and a wealth of fiber found in fruits and vegetables are crucial in nurturing the gut lining and fostering an environment conducive to healing and health. Some standout choices include:

- Berries: Strawberries, blueberries, and raspberries are loaded with antioxidants that support gut health.
- Leafy Greens: Spinach, kale, and Swiss chard offer vitamins and minerals vital for reducing inflammation.
- Bell Peppers and Tomatoes: Rich in vitamin C and antioxidants, they support the immune system and combat inflammation.

Incorporating a rainbow of fruits and vegetables into your daily meals makes your plate more appealing and ensures a broad spectrum of nutrients to support gut health.

Inclusion Strategies

Infusing your diet with anti-inflammatory foods can be both simple and delicious. Here are some practical tips to effortlessly integrate them into your daily meals:

- Smoothie Power: Start your day with a smoothie packed with leafy greens, berries, and a tablespoon of flaxseed or chia seeds. It's a convenient way to get a hefty dose of anti-inflammatory nutrients in one go.
- Salad Savvy: Make salads a staple of your lunch routine. Experiment with different greens, add some grilled salmon or tuna for omega-3s, and toss in various colorful vegetables. A drizzle of olive oil and a squeeze of lemon juice can enhance the anti-inflammatory benefits further.

- Snack Smart: Keep a stash of nuts, seeds, and fresh fruit for snacks. These are nutritious and help curb hunger with their fiber and healthy fats, steering you away from less healthy options.
- Diverse Dinners: Incorporate at least two different vegetables with your evening meal, and choose whole grains like quinoa or brown rice to accompany your omega-3-rich fish. The diversity in your diet will keep things exciting and ensure a wide range of anti-inflammatory benefits.

By embracing anti-inflammatory foods, you're not just feeding your taste buds; you're nourishing your gut and, by extension, your overall health. These dietary choices build a foundation for a robust digestive system capable of withstanding the challenges of modern living and nutritional habits. Remember, every meal is an opportunity to support your gut health, so choose wisely and enjoy the rich flavors and benefits these foods bring to your table.

3.3 PREBIOTICS AND PROBIOTICS: BALANCING YOUR GUT FLORA

The health of your gut microbiome is not just about the absence of harmful bacteria; it's equally about the presence and prosperity of beneficial ones. This is where prebiotics and probiotics come into play, acting as the nurturing gardeners of your gut's ecosystem, each with a specific role in encouraging a flourishing digestive tract.

Understanding Prebiotics and Probiotics

Prebiotics are the food that feeds the good bacteria in your gut, promoting their growth and activity. They are non-digestible fibers that pass through the upper part of the gastrointestinal tract and stimulate the growth or activity of advantageous bacteria that colonize the large bowel by acting as food for them.

On the other hand, probiotics are live beneficial bacteria introduced into the digestive system. They can help restore the natural balance of gut bacteria, enhancing health. Prebiotics and probiotics create a symbiotic relationship, fostering an environment conducive to gut health and well-being.

Natural Sources

Including prebiotics and probiotics in your diet doesn't require a complete overhaul but a mindful addition of certain foods rich in these beneficial components.

For Prebiotics, look to include:

- Garlic and onions: These everyday kitchen staples are not just for flavor. They are excellent sources of inulin, a type of prebiotic fiber.
- Bananas: Especially when they're a bit green, bananas are a good source of prebiotics.
- Asparagus: Another vegetable high in inulin, asparagus can be a tasty addition to your prebiotic diet.
- Barley and oats: Whole grains like these are heart-healthy and good sources of prebiotic fibers.

For Probiotics, consider adding:

- Yogurt is one of the best-known sources of probiotics. Look for labels that mention "live active cultures."
- Kefir: A fermented probiotic milk drink that's a richer source of live cultures compared to yogurt.
- Sauerkraut: Fermented cabbage not only provides probiotics but is also rich in vitamins C, B, and K.
- Kimchi: This spicy Korean side dish made from fermented vegetables brings a variety of probiotics and a punch of flavor.

Supplementation Considerations

While getting prebiotics and probiotics from food is ideal, supplementation may be necessary to achieve specific health goals or address digestive issues. Here's how to navigate the world of supplements:

- Quality Matters: Look for supplements from reputable brands that have been third-party tested for potency and purity.
- Probiotic Strains: Different strains of probiotics serve different purposes. For example, Lactobacillus acidophilus is often used for its digestive benefits, while Bifidobacterium bifidum can support the immune system.
- Prebiotic Supplements: These can be a good option if you struggle to get enough prebiotic fiber from your diet. Look for supplements containing inulin or FOS (fructooligosaccharides).

When considering supplements, it's always wise to consult with a healthcare professional, especially if you have underlying health conditions or are taking other medications.

Synergy for Gut Health

The interplay between prebiotics and probiotics is a dance of mutual benefit, enhancing each other's effectiveness in supporting gut health. This symbiotic relationship ensures that probiotics have the necessary nutrients to thrive, leading to a more balanced and resilient gut microbiome. Here's how you can harness their synergy:

- Combine Them in Meals: Adding banana slices to your yogurt or serving sauerkraut as a side dish to a meal rich in garlic and onions can maximize the prebiotic-probiotic benefits.
- Timing: While it's not crucial to consume prebiotics and probiotics together at every meal, incorporating a variety of both throughout your day can help maintain a healthy gut microbiome balance.
- Diversity is Key: Just as a diverse diet supports overall health, a variety of prebiotic and probiotic sources can enhance the diversity of your gut flora, contributing to a more vital, more robust gut ecosystem.

Nurturing your gut's flora through a thoughtful blend of prebiotics and probiotics aids digestion and sets the stage for a healthier, more vibrant self. The foods we eat can directly communicate with our gut bacteria, influencing our digestive health and overall well-being. By making room on your plate for these gut-friendly foods, you're taking a pivotal step towards a balanced microbiome and, consequently, a balanced life.

3.4 THE IMPORTANCE OF FIBER: TYPES, SOURCES, AND BENEFITS

In the tapestry of gut health, fiber stands out as a crucial thread, weaving through our digestive systems and offering many benefits. Fiber is not just about avoiding that sluggish feeling or keeping things moving; it plays a complex role in our overall health, particularly when nurturing our gut microbiome. Let's unravel the details, starting with the basics of fiber types, moving through their sources, and understanding their indispensable role in our diets.

Types of Fiber

Fiber is often categorized into two main types: soluble and insoluble. Each serves a distinct purpose within the digestive tract, acting uniquely to support our health.

- Soluble Fiber: This type of fiber dissolves in water to form a gel-like substance. It can help to slow down the digestion process, which in turn can aid in controlling blood sugar levels and reduce cholesterol. For the gut specifically, soluble fiber is a feast for the beneficial bacteria residing there, promoting their growth and activity.
- Insoluble Fiber: Unlike its soluble counterpart, insoluble fiber does not dissolve in water. It adds bulk to the stool and helps food pass more quickly through the stomach and intestines, aiding in regular bowel movements and preventing constipation.

Fiber-Rich Foods

Finding natural sources of both fiber types is easy with a diet rich in whole foods. Here's where you can find these fibrous treasures:

For Soluble Fiber:

- Legumes such as beans, lentils, and peas are high in protein and excellent sources of soluble fiber.
- Oats and barley bring a comforting texture and are perfect for starting the day with a gut-friendly boost.
- Fruits like apples, oranges, and pears, with their skins on, offer a sweet way to incorporate soluble fiber into your diet.

For Insoluble Fiber:

- Whole grains, including whole wheat flour, wheat bran, and brown rice, provide a hearty meal base.
- Vegetables, notably carrots, cucumbers, and tomatoes, add crunch and fiber to any dish.
- Nuts and seeds are not just for snacking; they're also a crunchy source of insoluble fiber.

Fiber Intake Guidelines

The question of how much fiber we need can lead to some confusion. The general recommendation is about 25 grams daily for women and 38 grams for men. However, the reality is that most people don't reach these numbers. Increasing your fiber intake too quickly can lead to discomfort, so it's wise to do it gradually. Here's how:

- Start by adding just one or two high-fiber foods to your diet each week, allowing your body to adjust.
- Drink plenty of water. As you increase your fiber intake, water is essential to help fiber do its job and prevent constipation.
- Spread your fiber intake throughout the day, incorporating fibrous foods into each meal and snack.

Fiber's Role in Microbiome Health

The benefits of fiber extend well beyond digestion and regularity. Fiber acts as a prebiotic, serving as food for the beneficial bacteria in the gut. This relationship fosters a flourishing microbiome, which supports a healthy immune system, enhances nutrient absorption, and even influences mood regulation.

Fiber breakdown by these gut bacteria produces short-chain fatty acids (SCFAs), compounds with anti-inflammatory properties that can strengthen the gut barrier function. This not only helps in warding off unwanted pathogens but also plays a role in preventing conditions like obesity, type 2 diabetes, and colorectal cancer.

Incorporating various fibrous foods into your diet ensures that your microbiome receives a broad spectrum of prebiotics, promoting diversity among the bacterial species. This diversity is vital to a resilient digestive system, capable of withstanding and recovering from disruptions such as antibiotic use or a bout of illness.

Focusing on fiber is a step in the right direction for those looking to enhance their gut health. It's not merely about adding a sprinkle of bran to your morning yogurt or swapping white rice for brown. It's about embracing a diet that celebrates whole foods, respects the body's need for gradual change, and recognizes the profound impact of diet on our microbiome. Through mindful inclusion of both soluble and insoluble fibers, we nourish not just our bodies but the entire ecosystem residing within, paving the way for lasting health and vitality.

3.5 INTEGRATING FERMENTED FOODS: A PRACTICAL APPROACH

In the quest for optimal gut health, fermented foods stand out as both ancient allies and modern friends. Through fermentation, these foods become enriched with probiotics, beneficial bacteria that play a pivotal role in maintaining a healthy gut microbiome. The beauty of incorporating fermented foods into one's diet lies in their health benefits and the depth and complexity of flavors they introduce to our meals.

Fermented foods bring a wealth of diversity to our gut, encouraging the proliferation of good bacteria and enhancing the resilience of our microbiome. This, in turn, has been linked to improved digestion, enhanced immune function, and even a positive impact on mental health. Fermentation also increases the availability of vitamins and minerals in these foods, making them even more beneficial.

A delightful variety of fermented foods can be found across cultures worldwide. Here are a few to consider:

- Yogurt and Kefir: Dairy-based but transformed through fermentation, these are rich in probiotics. Opt for versions without added sugar to maximize benefits.

- Sauerkraut: Fermented cabbage, known for its tangy flavor, is a staple in many Eastern European cuisines. It's not only a probiotic powerhouse but also a good source of fiber.
- Kombucha is a fermented tea that has gained popularity for its fizzy bite and health-promoting properties. To enjoy its full benefits, ensure it's low in sugar.
- Kimchi: A Korean favorite, this spicy, fermented vegetable mix often includes cabbage and radishes, offering a flavorful way to support your gut health.
- Miso: A Japanese seasoning made from fermented soybeans, rich in flavor and probiotics. It's a versatile ingredient for soups, marinades, and dressings.

Incorporating these fermented delights into your daily diet can be easy and enjoyable. Here are some creative and practical tips:

- Start your day with a bowl of yogurt, adding a sprinkle of nuts and fresh fruit for a gut-friendly breakfast.
- Swap out traditional condiments for sauerkraut or kimchi, adding them to sandwiches, salads, or as a side to your main meal for an extra probiotic punch.
- Experiment with kombucha as a refreshing alternative to sugary drinks, enjoying its unique taste and gut health benefits.
- Use miso to deepen the flavor of soups and sauces, introducing probiotics and a rich, savory taste to your dishes.

For those inclined towards culinary adventures, fermenting at home is a rewarding practice that connects us to traditional food preparation methods. Starting with simple recipes can demystify the process and open up a world of fermentation possibilities. Consider these beginner-friendly ideas:

- Homemade Sauerkraut: With just cabbage, salt, and time, you can create your batch of sauerkraut, controlling the level of tanginess to your preference.
- Easy Kefir: You can ferment your kefir by obtaining kefir grains and adding them to milk. You can enjoy it plain or as a base for smoothies.
- Quick Pickles: Cucumbers, carrots, or radishes can be quickly pickled in a brine solution, offering a crunchy, probiotic-rich snack or garnish.

Engaging in fermentation enriches your diet with probiotics. It fosters a connection to the food you eat, enhancing your appreciation for the role of bacteria in our health and well-being.

As we wrap up this exploration into fermented foods, it becomes evident that these traditional staples offer more than just flavor; they provide a direct route to nurturing our gut health. By embracing the diversity of fermented foods available, experimenting with incorporating them into our meals, and even venturing into home fermentation, we can support our microbiome deliciously and satisfyingly. This approach to diet focused on variety, flavor, and the health-promoting properties of food lays a strong foundation for a healthy gut and a vibrant, thriving self.

As we move forward, let's remember that our dietary choices have profound implications for our health. By choosing wisely, we can support our body's natural systems in their essential work, onwards to a healthier, happier gut.

SPECIAL DIETS AND THEIR ROLE IN GUT HEALTH

Navigating the world of special diets can feel like decoding a complex map with multiple paths, each promising a destination of improved gut health. Yet, only some paths are suitable for everyone. Understanding the nuances of each diet, the science behind them, and how they interact with our bodies can turn this map into a valuable tool for finding the route that aligns with our unique digestive landscapes.

4.1 THE GLUTEN-FREE LIFESTYLE: BEYOND CELIAC DISEASE

Non-Celiac Gluten Sensitivity

While celiac disease has long been recognized, another condition, non-celiac gluten sensitivity (NCGS), has emerged, broadening the spectrum of gluten-related disorders. Unlike celiac disease, where gluten consumption damages the small intestine, NCGS involves a range of symptoms in the absence of celiac disease and wheat allergy. Symptoms often include bloating, gas, diarrhea, and even non-digestive issues such as brain fog and fatigue, triggering discomfort without the intestinal damage seen in celiac disease.

For those dealing with NCGS, removing gluten from the diet has shown significant symptom relief. The key here is vigilance; gluten hides in many foods where you wouldn't expect it, making label reading a crucial skill.

Nutritional Considerations

While a gluten-free diet is beneficial for those with gluten sensitivities, it also risks nutritional deficiencies. Whole grains, a common source of gluten, are also rich in B vitamins, fiber, and iron. Removing them without careful planning can lead to gaps in nutrition.

To counteract this, focusing on naturally gluten-free whole foods ensures a nutrient-dense diet. Quinoa, brown rice, and buckwheat are excellent grain alternatives that provide the fiber and vitamins missing from refined gluten-free products. Incorporating a variety of fruits, vegetables, lean proteins, and healthy fats can cover the nutritional bases, supporting overall health and well-being.

Whole Foods Focus

Emphasizing whole, naturally gluten-free foods not only addresses the nutritional challenges of a gluten-free diet but also simplifies it. Rather than navigating the often confusing and expensive world of gluten-free substitutes, filling your plate with unprocessed foods eliminates the guesswork. Think colorful salads, hearty soups, and stir-fries packed with vegetables, lean meats, and gluten-free grains.

Label Reading Skills

Gluten can lurk in places you'd least expect, from sauces and soups to processed meats and some medications. Becoming proficient at reading labels is essential for maintaining a truly gluten-free diet. Here are a few tips:

- Look for a gluten-free certification on products. This ensures the food meets strict standards for gluten content.
- Familiarize yourself with common sources of hidden gluten, such as malt flavoring, modified food starch, and certain food additives.
- Be cautious with products labeled "wheat-free"; they may still contain gluten from other sources.
- Contact the manufacturer to clarify a product's gluten content when in doubt.

Transitioning to a gluten-free lifestyle, especially for those with NCGS, doesn't have to be a daunting overhaul of your diet. You can confidently navigate this path by focusing on whole foods, understanding potential nutritional gaps, and honing your label-reading skills. The goal is to eliminate gluten and create a balanced and nourishing diet that supports your gut health and overall wellness.

4.2 THE LOW-FODMAP JOURNEY: NAVIGATING DIGESTIVE RELIEF

The low-FODMAP diet emerges as a beacon of hope for many in the realm of dietary strategies for managing irritable bowel syndrome (IBS) and similar gastrointestinal discomforts. This diet, grounded in reducing certain fermentable carbohydrates, has been scientifically shown to alleviate common symptoms associated with digestive distress.

The acronym FODMAP stands for fermentable oligosaccharides, disaccharides, monosaccharides, and polyols, short-chain carbohydrates that the small intestine absorbs poorly. When these carbohydrates ferment in the gut, they can cause gas, bloating, and other IBS symptoms. The low-FODMAP diet aims to minimize the intake of foods high in these substances, relieving many individuals.

Phases of Low-FODMAP Dieting

The low-FODMAP diet unfolds in three structured phases, each crucial for understanding and managing one's response to various foods.

- Elimination: This initial phase involves removing high-FODMAP foods from the diet for a period, typically 4-6 weeks. The goal is to reset the gut and observe whether symptoms improve without these triggers.
- Reintroduction: Following the elimination phase, high-FODMAP foods are methodically reintroduced into the diet one group at a time. This careful process allows individuals to pinpoint which specific FODMAPs trigger their symptoms.
- Personalization: The final phase focuses on creating a long-term, sustainable diet based on the findings from the reintroduction phase. This personalized diet includes as wide a variety of foods as possible while managing and minimizing IBS symptoms.

Common Challenges

Adopting and adhering to the low-FODMAP diet presents several challenges and misconceptions that can hinder progress.

- Restrictive Nature: The diet's initial restrictive phase can feel daunting and may lead to feelings of dietary deprivation. It's vital to remember this phase is temporary and exploratory.
- Misunderstanding the Goal: Some might mistakenly view the low-FODMAP diet as a lifelong dietary change rather than a temporary investigative tool. The aim is to reintroduce as many foods as possible without triggering symptoms, not permanently eliminating them.
- Overlooking Nutritional Balance: Given the diet's restrictive phase, nutritional deficiencies can occur if not properly managed. Ensuring a balanced intake of nutrients is crucial throughout this dietary approach.

Maintaining Nutritional Balance

Ensuring a nutritionally rich diet while navigating the low-FODMAP landscape requires thoughtful planning and creativity. Here are some strategies to maintain nutritional balance:

- Diverse Food Selection: Focus on incorporating a broad range of low-FODMAP fruits, vegetables, grains, proteins, and fats to ensure a well-rounded diet. This diversity helps cover essential vitamins and minerals that might be lacking due to eliminating certain foods.

- Mindful Meal Planning: Prepare meals that are low in FODMAPs and nutritionally dense. For example, a dinner plate could include a serving of grilled chicken, a side of quinoa, and a variety of low-FODMAP vegetables like carrots and zucchini.
- Supplement Wisely: In cases where dietary restrictions limit the intake of certain nutrients, consider supplements to fill the gaps. Key focus areas include fiber, calcium, and vitamin D. Consulting with a healthcare professional before starting supplements ensures safe and appropriate choices.
- Seek Professional Guidance: Working with a dietitian familiar with the low-FODMAP diet can provide personalized advice on meeting nutritional needs while following the diet's phases. They can offer tailored meal plans, suggest suitable supplements, and provide support throughout the dieting process.

By navigating the low-FODMAP diet with an emphasis on personalization, mindful reintroduction of foods, and a commitment to nutritional balance, individuals can discover a dietary pattern that supports their gut health without compromising their nutritional well-being. This approach alleviates symptoms and promotes a positive relationship with food, grounded in understanding and mindfulness.

4.3 THE KETOGENIC DIET: IMPACTS ON THE GUT MICROBIOME

In recent years, the ketogenic diet has surged in popularity, touted for its potential to prompt significant weight loss and manage various health conditions. This high-fat, moderate-protein, and very low-carbohydrate diet shifts the body's metabolism away from carbs and towards fat and ketones.

Keto Basics

Under normal circumstances, the body utilizes carbohydrates as its primary fuel source. The ketogenic diet drastically reduces carbohydrate intake, forcing the body into ketosis, where fat is burned for energy instead of carbs. This metabolic shift affects energy usage and various bodily systems, including the gut microbiome.

Gut Microbiome Changes

Emerging research suggests that adopting a ketogenic diet can lead to notable changes in the gut microbiome's composition. Specifically, studies have observed an increase in the abundance of certain bacteria, such as Akkermansia muciniphila, known for its beneficial effects on metabolic health. Conversely, there's a decrease in the diversity of the gut flora, which could affect gut health. Reducing fiber-rich food intake, a consequence of limiting carbohydrates might reduce gut bacteria associated with fiber metabolism.

- Akkermansia muciniphila has been linked to improved metabolic markers and increased intestinal lining thickness, potentially offering protective effects against obesity and type 2 diabetes.
- Reducing fiber-dependent bacteria could impact the production of short-chain fatty acids (SCFAs), compounds critical for colon health and immune function.

Potential Benefits and Drawbacks

While the ketogenic diet offers promising weight loss and blood sugar control benefits, its long-term effects on gut health warrant careful consideration. On the one hand, the increase in beneficial bacteria like Akkermansia suggests potential positive impacts on metabolic health and possibly even protection against certain diseases.

However, the decreased microbial diversity and diminished populations of fiber-fermenting bacteria highlight potential drawbacks. A diverse gut microbiome is generally considered a hallmark of good gut health, associated with a lower risk of chronic diseases and improved immune function. Reduced SCFA production due to less fiber fermentation could decrease colon health over time.

Personalization and Moderation

Given the ketogenic diet's impact on the gut microbiome, those considering this dietary approach might benefit from strategies that mitigate potential adverse effects while leveraging its benefits:

- Incorporate gut-friendly, low-carb vegetables: Non-starchy vegetables like leafy greens, broccoli, and cauliflower are low in carbs but high in fiber, vitamins, and minerals. Including a variety of these in the diet can help support a healthy gut microbiome by providing prebiotic fiber to feed beneficial bacteria.
- Consider a cyclical approach: Some individuals may find a cyclical ketogenic diet, which involves periods of higher carb intake, allows for greater flexibility and easier inclusion of a wider variety of plant-based foods. This approach can help maintain microbial diversity by reintroducing fiber-rich carbs supporting gut bacteria.
- Focus on high-quality fats: Choosing sources of healthy fats, such as avocados, nuts, seeds, and olive oil, can help reduce inflammation and support gut health. Avoiding overly processed fats and oils is crucial to prevent adverse impacts on gut and overall health.
- Supplement strategically: Given the reduction in certain food groups, supplementing with fiber and probiotics could help support gut health. Soluble fiber supplements, in particular, can help compensate for the lower intake of fiber-rich foods, supporting SCFA production and bowel regularity.
- Monitor and adjust: It is essential to pay close attention to how the body responds to a ketogenic diet. If digestive issues arise, changing the approach to include more prebiotic-rich foods or considering a less restrictive low-carb diet may be beneficial. Consulting with a healthcare professional experienced in nutritional and gut health can provide guidance tailored to individual needs and goals.

While the ketogenic diet presents a promising option for weight loss and metabolic health improvement, understanding its potential impacts on the gut microbiome is crucial for making informed dietary choices. Balancing the benefits with potential drawbacks involves careful planning and personalization, ensuring that gut health is preserved and promoted even when carbohydrates are significantly reduced. Through strategic dietary adjustments and mindful monitoring, individuals can navigate the ketogenic landscape in a way that supports both their metabolic and gut health objectives.

4.4 VEGAN AND VEGETARIAN DIETS: PROS AND CONS FOR GUT HEALTH

Turning our attention to plant-based diets, it's clear that shifting away from animal products towards a more vegetable-centric plate has implications for our gut microbiome, among other health aspects. Vegan and vegetarian diets, rich in fruits, vegetables, legumes, and grains, naturally promote a diverse and vibrant gut flora community. This diversity is a cornerstone of gut health, associated with better nutrient absorption, improved digestion, and a reduced risk of chronic illnesses.

However, embarking on a vegan or vegetarian lifestyle requires mindful planning to ensure that all nutritional needs are met, given the exclusion of meat and other animal products. Here's a closer look at the dynamics of plant-based diets in the context of gut health and overall well-being.

Impact on Gut Health

Plant-based diets bring a banquet of benefits to the gut's microbial community. The high intake of diverse plant fibers fuels beneficial bacteria, fostering a robust and diverse microbiome. Studies have shown that those following a vegan or vegetarian diet tend to have more protective species linked to reduced inflammation and lower disease risk. These diets are naturally high in polyphenols, compounds found in fruits and vegetables, which act as antioxidants and further support gut health by promoting the growth of beneficial bacteria.

Nutritional Considerations

While the advantages for gut health are significant, vegan and vegetarian diets do pose potential challenges in meeting specific nutritional needs:

- Vitamin B12: Primarily found in animal products, B12 is crucial for nerve function and DNA and red blood cell production. Vegans and vegetarians must seek alternative sources, such as fortified foods or supplements, to avoid deficiencies.
- Iron: While plant foods contain iron, it's in a form that's less readily absorbed by the body. Including vitamin C-rich foods in meals can enhance iron absorption from plant sources.
- Omega-3 Fatty Acids: Essential for brain health, omega-3s are primarily found in fatty fish. Flaxseeds, chia seeds, walnuts, and algae-based supplements can provide these essential fats in a plant-based diet.

- Calcium and Vitamin D: Crucial for bone health, these nutrients can be found in fortified plant milk and juices, leafy green vegetables, and by ensuring adequate sun exposure for vitamin D synthesis.

Fiber Advantage

A standout feature of vegan and vegetarian diets is their high fiber content, not just in volume but in variety. This abundance of fiber has multifaceted benefits for gut health:

- Promotes Regularity: A high-fiber diet helps maintain regular bowel movements and prevent constipation by increasing stool bulk and speeding up transit time.
- Feeds Good Bacteria: Different types of fiber serve as prebiotics, nourishing beneficial gut bacteria and enabling them to produce health-promoting short-chain fatty acids.
- Supports Weight Management: High-fiber foods are more filling, which can help control appetite and manage weight, indirectly benefiting gut health by reducing the risk of obesity-related complications.

Balanced Plant-Based Eating

Adopting a plant-based diet that nurtures gut health while ensuring nutritional adequacy involves more than simply cutting out animal products. It requires a strategic approach to meal planning:

- Varied Protein Sources: Incorporate a mix of plant

proteins from beans, lentils, tofu, tempeh, and quinoa to ensure a complete amino acid profile.
- Whole Foods: Prioritize whole, unprocessed plant foods to maximize nutrient intake and minimize exposure to additives that could disrupt the gut microbiome.
- Fermented Plant Foods: Include vegan sources of probiotics like sauerkraut, kimchi, miso, and plant-based yogurts to introduce beneficial bacteria into the gut.
- Mindful Supplementation: Consider supplements for nutrients that are challenging to obtain from plant-based foods alone, such as B12 and omega-3 fatty acids, after consulting with a healthcare provider.

Vegan and vegetarian diets can be healthfully and deliciously adapted to support gut health by emphasizing variety, whole foods, and mindful supplementation. This approach caters to the gut's microbial needs and aligns with broader health goals, offering a comprehensive strategy for wellness that extends beyond the digestive system.

4.5 ELIMINATION DIETS: FINDING WHAT WORKS FOR YOU

Identifying the foods that don't agree with your digestive system can sometimes feel like solving a complex puzzle with pieces that don't quite fit. That's where elimination diets step in, a helpful tool in this detective work. By methodically removing and reintroducing specific foods, you gain insights into which foods may be causing issues such as bloating, gas, or even more severe reactions.

Purpose of Elimination Diets

The primary goal of an elimination diet is to pinpoint food sensitivities and intolerances that might be stealthily impacting your gut health. Unlike food allergies, which are typically immediate and potentially life-threatening reactions to foods, sensitivities, and intolerances can have subtler, delayed effects, making them harder to identify. By cutting out certain foods and monitoring symptoms for changes, you can discover which foods your body might react to.

Conducting an Elimination Diet

Embarking on this diet requires a structured approach:

1. Choose What to Eliminate: Commonly, the diet starts by removing foods known to be frequent irritants, such as dairy, gluten, soy, eggs, and nuts. Your choices might vary based on your suspicions of what's causing discomfort.
2. Plan Your Meals: After eliminating the selected foods from your diet, plan your meals around what's left. This might seem limiting initially, but it's an opportunity to explore new dishes and flavors.
3. Monitor Symptoms: During this phase, keep a detailed food diary, noting what you eat and any symptoms you experience. This record is crucial for identifying patterns between food consumption and digestive distress.
4. Duration: Typically, this elimination phase lasts about 2-4 weeks, allowing enough time for any improvements in symptoms to become apparent.

Reintroduction Phase

This phase is about slowly reintroducing the eliminated foods back into your diet, one at a time, while observing for any symptoms. Each food should be reintroduced over a few days, with a return to the elimination diet in between, to clear the system and ready it for the next test. This careful process helps isolate which foods are problematic.

Long-Term Strategy

Remember, elimination diets are not meant to be permanent. They're a diagnostic tool, not a lifestyle. Once you've identified foods that cause issues, you can:

- Avoid or Limit Problem Foods: Knowing your triggers allows you to avoid or limit these foods, potentially relieving your symptoms.
- Seek Alternatives: For every food that causes discomfort, there's often an alternative that doesn't. Discovering these can diversify your diet and introduce you to new favorites.
- Balance and Variety: Post-elimination, aim for a varied and balanced diet, ensuring you get all the nutrients your body needs without the foods that cause you distress.

This approach helps manage gut health issues and contributes to a broader understanding of how different foods affect your body, empowering you to make informed dietary choices.

In wrapping up, the journey through elimination diets shines a light on food's powerful impact on our gut health and overall well-being. By identifying the foods that do not sit well with us and understanding how to navigate our diets accordingly, we take a significant step towards better digestive health and quality of life. The insights gained from this process underscore the importance of listening to our bodies and responding with care. As we move forward, remember the value of such mindfulness in all health and wellness, readying us for the next steps in our quest for well-being.

UNRAVELING THE STRESS-GUT CONNECTION

Imagine your gut as a serene garden, where each microbe is a harmonious plant. Now, envision stress as a storm wreaking havoc on this peaceful landscape. This imagery isn't just poetic; it reflects stress's impact on our gut health. With its fast pace and high demands, modern life often brings more stress storms than our gut garden can handle. Here, we'll explore how stress influences gut health and practical ways to shield our internal garden from these storms.

5.1 THE VICIOUS CYCLE: STRESS, CORTISOL, AND YOUR GUT

When stress kicks in, your body doesn't take it lightly. It responds by releasing cortisol, a hormone designed to help you cope in the short term. However, when stress becomes a constant visitor, elevated cortisol levels can disrupt your gut, leading to inflammation and a host of digestive issues. Think of cortisol as fertilizer that's good in small amounts but harmful in excess.

Chronic stress doesn't just stop there. It can alter your gut microbiota composition, leading to an increased risk of gastrointestinal disorders. Imagine each stressful event as a wave washing over your gut garden, each time eroding a bit more of the protective barrier and allowing harmful bacteria to take root.

Breaking the Cycle

To protect your gut garden from these stress storms, consider the following strategies:

- Mindfulness and Breathing Exercises: These are your tools to calm the storm. Deep breathing or focusing on the present moment can significantly reduce stress levels. Try starting your day with a five-minute breathing exercise, focusing solely on the rhythm of your breath. This practice can set a tranquil tone for the day, shielding your gut from stress-induced turmoil.
- Lifestyle Adjustments: Incorporating regular exercise, ensuring adequate sleep, and engaging in hobbies can act as barriers against stress. Regular physical activity, for instance, not only decreases cortisol levels but also promotes a healthy gut microbiome. Aim for activities you enjoy, whether a brisk walk in the park, a dance class, or gardening. Find joy in these activities, and let them be your sanctuary from stress.

Recognizing Stress Signals

Identifying early signs of stress is crucial in preventing its adverse effects on gut health. These signals can range from irritability and fatigue to changes in appetite or sleep patterns. You can deploy your stress-reduction tools before the storm hits full force by staying vigilant.

- Keep a Stress Diary: For a week, jot down moments when you feel stressed, including what triggered it and how you responded. This record can reveal patterns and help you develop more effective coping strategies.
- Set Realistic Expectations: Often, stress stems from overcommitting or setting unrealistic standards for ourselves. Adjusting our expectations and learning to say no can reduce unnecessary stressors that threaten our gut health.

Practical stress management steps are avoiding discomfort and cultivating a thriving internal ecosystem. By implementing these strategies, you can create a resilient gut garden capable of withstanding the storms of modern life.

5.2 MEDITATION AND MINDFULNESS: TOOLS FOR STRESS REDUCTION

In today's fast-paced world, ancient meditation and mindfulness practices offer a sanctuary for the mind and the gut. These practices, rooted in centuries-old traditions, have gained recognition in the wellness community for their profound benefits on mental clarity, emotional balance, and digestive health. Meditation and mindfulness, at their core, encourage a state of presence and awareness, counterbalancing daily life's hustle and stress.

Introduction to Mindfulness

Mindfulness is being fully present and engaged in the moment, aware of our thoughts and feelings without getting caught up in them. This simple yet powerful technique can transform how we relate to experiences, reducing stress and its harmful effects on the gut. Research suggests that mindfulness can lower cortisol levels, easing the inflammatory responses in the gut that stress can exacerbate. By fostering a calm mental environment, mindfulness may also enhance the diversity and resilience of our gut microbiome, contributing to overall digestive well-being.

Practical Meditation Techniques

Incorporating meditation into your daily routine doesn't require hours of silent contemplation. Even a few minutes can make a difference. Here are some practical techniques to get you started:

- Focused Attention Meditation: Sit quietly and focus on your breath, a word, or a mantra. When your mind wanders, gently bring your focus back. This practice can help train your attention and reduce stress.
- Body Scan Meditation: Lie down and mentally scan your body from head to toe, noting any sensations without judgment. This technique is excellent for releasing tension and fostering bodily awareness.
- Walking Meditation: Find a quiet path and walk slowly, fully immersed in the experience of walking, noting the sensation of each step. This form can be particularly appealing for those who find peace in movement.

Each technique serves as a tool to quiet the mind, offering respite from the barrage of thoughts and worries that can fuel stress and disrupt our digestive processes.

Mindful Eating

At the intersection of mindfulness and nourishment lies the practice of mindful eating. This approach to food is about fully experiencing the act of eating, from the flavors and textures of the food to the sensations of fullness. Mindful eating encourages a deep connection with our meals, transforming eating into a routine and nourishing experience. Here's how it can positively impact digestive health:

- Enhances Digestion: Slowing down and thoroughly chewing your food aids digestion, making it easier for your gut to absorb nutrients.
- Promotes Satiety: Tuning into hunger and fullness signals can prevent overeating, supporting a healthy gut and weight.
- Reduces Stress Eating: Mindful eating helps break the cycle of emotional eating by fostering an awareness of why and how we eat.

Incorporating mindful eating into your life can start with small steps, like eliminating distractions during meals or taking a moment to express gratitude for your food. These acts of mindfulness enrich the eating experience and support a harmonious digestive system.

Building a Regular Practice

Establishing a consistent mindfulness and meditation practice can seem daunting amidst the demands of daily life. Yet, the key to success lies in simplicity and routine. Here are strategies to build and maintain a practice:

- Start Small: Begin with just five minutes a day. Once this feels manageable, gradually increase the duration.
- Set a Regular Time: Whether first thing in the morning or during a lunch break, having a set time for your practice can help it become a natural part of your day.
- Create a Dedicated Space: Designate a quiet, comfortable spot in your home for meditation. This can be a simple corner with a cushion or chair, free from distractions.
- Embrace Patience: Progress in meditation and mindfulness is subtle. Rather than striving for a particular outcome, focus on the practice itself, knowing the benefits will unfold in time.
- Use Resources: Countless apps, books, and online courses can guide you through the nuances of these practices. Find tools that resonate with you and use them to enrich your journey.

In facing the everyday challenges of building a regular practice, such as time constraints or fluctuating motivation, remember that each moment of mindfulness is a step towards a more balanced mind and gut. The beauty of these practices lies in their flexibility and accessibility; they can be tailored to fit into any lifestyle, offering a refuge of calm in the storm of daily stress. Through meditation and mindful eating, we cultivate a serene mind and nurture a resilient digestive system, unlocking a synergy of wellness that radiates throughout our entire being.

5.3 SLEEP'S ROLE IN GUT HEALTH: CONNECTING THE DOTS

The intricate dance between sleep and gut health is fascinating, where each step and turn affects the other profoundly. At the heart of this relationship is the understanding that our gut health doesn't operate in isolation; it's deeply influenced by our sleep patterns. When we cut corners on rest, it's not just our energy levels that take a hit—our microbiome feels the brunt, too. Sleep disruptions can lead to noticeable shifts in the composition of our gut flora, potentially paving the way for digestive discomfort and weakened immune responses. Essentially, when our sleep suffers, our gut does too.

Navigating the complexities of this relationship starts with recognizing that inadequate sleep can lead to an imbalance in the gut microbiome. This imbalance can increase susceptibility to conditions like obesity, type 2 diabetes, and even mood disorders. The multifaceted mechanisms include changes in appetite-regulating hormones, increased stress levels, and direct impacts on the gut's bacterial composition. To foster a healthy gut, prioritizing quality sleep is as critical as choosing the right foods.

Improving Sleep Hygiene

Creating an environment conducive to restful sleep can significantly enhance both the quantity and quality of sleep. Here are actionable steps to refine your sleep hygiene:

- Establish a Regular Sleep Schedule: Going to bed and waking up at the same time every day sets your body's internal clock, making it easier to fall asleep and wake up naturally.
- Craft a Restful Environment: Ensure your bedroom is cool, quiet, and dark. Use blackout curtains, earplugs, or white noise machines to block out disturbances.
- Limit Screen Time: The blue light emitted by screens can interfere with your body's ability to prepare for sleep. Try switching off electronic devices at least an hour before bedtime.
- Wind-Down Routine: Develop a pre-sleep ritual that helps your body transition into sleep mode. This might include reading, gentle stretching, or a warm bath.

Impact of Sleep Disorders

Sleep disorders like insomnia not only rob you of rest but can also exacerbate gut health issues. The stress of lying awake can trigger digestive symptoms, while the lack of restorative sleep can alter the gut's bacterial balance. If you're struggling with a sleep disorder, seeking professional guidance is vital. A healthcare provider can offer tailored advice and treatment options, ranging from cognitive-behavioral therapy for insomnia (CBT-I) to appropriate medication under supervision. Addressing sleep disorders is a crucial step in safeguarding both your rest and your gut health.

Natural Sleep Aids

For those seeking gentle ways to encourage sleep, several natural remedies and practices can offer support:

- Herbal Teas: Sipping on a warm cup of herbal tea, such as chamomile or lavender, before bed can be soothing and help ease you into sleep. These herbs are known for their relaxing properties.
- Relaxation Techniques: Deep breathing exercises or progressive muscle relaxation can help calm the mind and body, making it easier to drift off to sleep.
- Essential Oils: Aromatherapy using oils like lavender or valerian may promote relaxation and improve sleep quality. Consider adding a few drops to your bath or using a diffuser in your bedroom.
- Magnesium Supplements: Known as the relaxation mineral, magnesium plays a role in supporting deep, restorative sleep. Incorporating magnesium-rich foods into your diet or discussing supplementation with a healthcare provider could be beneficial.

Nurturing the sleep-gut connection reveals that fostering good sleep hygiene, addressing sleep disorders, and exploring natural sleep aids are not just steps toward better rest—they're integral to maintaining a healthy, balanced gut. As we navigate the challenges of modern life, paying attention to this interconnected relationship offers a path to improved digestive health and a more balanced, vibrant state of well-being.

5.4 EXERCISE AND GUT HEALTH: FINDING THE RIGHT BALANCE

Moving our bodies isn't just about staying fit or losing weight; it profoundly affects our internal ecosystem, particularly our gut. Regular physical activity has been shown to enrich the diversity of our gut bacteria, a critical factor in overall gut health. This diversity is crucial, as it helps improve digestion, boosts our immune system, and even affects our mood and energy levels. However, not all exercises are created equal, especially regarding gut health. Let's explore how to strike the right balance with physical activity to support, not strain, our digestive system.

The Benefits of Regular Exercise on Gut Health

Physical activity can significantly impact the makeup of our gut microbiota, promoting an increase in beneficial bacteria varieties. These bacteria play a vital role in breaking down food, absorbing nutrients, and protecting against harmful organisms. Moreover, exercise stimulates muscle movements that help propel food through the digestive system, reducing the likelihood of constipation and promoting regular bowel movements.

- Boosts Microbial Diversity: Engaging in consistent physical activity encourages the growth of a wide range of beneficial bacteria in the gut.
- Enhances Digestion and Absorption: Exercise improves the efficiency of the digestive process, allowing for better nutrient uptake and less bloating or discomfort after meals.

Finding the Right Exercise Type

The key to harnessing the benefits of exercise without overburdening our bodies lies in selecting the right type and intensity of activity. This choice is deeply personal and should consider your current fitness level, any existing health conditions, and how your body responds to different forms of exercise.

- Listen to Your Body: Pay attention to how you feel during and after exercise. Discomfort or prolonged fatigue may indicate that you need to adjust the type or intensity of your activity.
- Mix It Up: Incorporating various exercises can prevent boredom, reduce the risk of injury, and ensure a well-rounded approach to physical fitness. Consider combining cardiovascular exercises, strength training, and flexibility workouts.

Exercise and Digestion

While exercise generally promotes gut health, timing matters, especially when eating around your workouts. Eating a large meal right before intense physical activity can lead to digestive discomfort, as your body diverts blood flow away from the digestive system to support your muscles.

- Timing Meals: Aim to eat a light meal or snack that's easy to digest, about one to two hours before exercising. This can provide you with energy without causing digestive upset.
- Stay Hydrated: Adequate hydration is crucial for digestion

and can help prevent constipation. Ensure you're drinking enough water before, during, and after exercise.
- Post-Workout Nutrition: After exercising, focus on replenishing your body with a balanced meal that includes carbohydrates, protein, and fats to aid recovery and support gut health.

Low-Impact Options

Low-impact exercises can be especially beneficial for those dealing with digestive issues or looking for gentler ways to incorporate physical activity into their routine. These forms of exercise minimize stress on the body while providing the health benefits associated with regular movement.

- Yoga: Not only does yoga reduce stress, which can positively impact gut health, but certain poses are specifically designed to aid digestion. Poses that involve twisting can help stimulate digestive organs, promoting food movement through the digestive tract.
- Walking: A simple yet effective exercise, walking can be easily adapted to fit any fitness level. Regular walks help regulate bowel movements and are gentle on the digestive system.
- Swimming: This low-impact exercise provides a full-body workout without straining the joints or the digestive system. The rhythmic nature of swimming can also be calming, reducing stress levels and their negative impact on gut health.

- Cycling: Whether stationary or on a bike outdoors, cycling is another excellent low-impact option that supports cardiovascular health without stressing the digestive system. Adjusting the intensity allows you to control the level of exertion, making it suitable for various fitness levels.

Incorporating regular physical activity into your routine is a cornerstone of maintaining a healthy gut. You can support your digestive system without overexerting yourself by choosing the right type of exercise, paying attention to the timing of meals, and opting for low-impact activities when necessary. Remember, the goal is to enhance your health and well-being, creating a balanced approach that nurtures your body and gut.

5.5 TIME MANAGEMENT: REDUCING STRESS FOR BETTER DIGESTIVE HEALTH

When our days are packed with personal and professional tasks, the stress can quietly seep into our lives, often without notice until our gut health signals distress. The chaos of poorly managed time doesn't just steal our peace; it directly impacts our digestive wellness. Finding harmony in our schedules isn't about doing more; it's about strategic planning to ensure our well-being remains a priority.

The Silent Culprit: Poor Time Management

It's a subtle connection that often goes unnoticed, but the link between how we manage our time and our gut health is unmistakably strong. When overwhelmed, our body responds by ramping up stress levels, leading to a cascade of digestive issues, from indigestion to more severe gut-related conditions. It's a cycle that starts with the clock and ends with our health. Recognizing this relationship is the first step toward creating a lifestyle that supports, rather than undermines, our digestive wellness.

Crafting a Priority List

The art of prioritizing tasks is akin to preparing a well-balanced meal—it requires thoughtful consideration of what's essential and what can wait. Here's how to approach your to-do list to alleviate the feeling of being overwhelmed:

- Start by listing all your tasks, both big and small.
- Mark each task with a level of urgency and importance. Those that are both urgent and important should take precedence.
- Learn to identify tasks that, although they may seem pressing, have little impact on your overall goals or well-being. These can often be delegated or dropped altogether.

This approach clears your schedule and mind, reducing stress directly affecting your gut health.

Boundaries: The Foundation of Time Management

Setting boundaries is crucial in maintaining a healthy balance between work, personal life, and wellness. It's about knowing when to say yes and, more importantly, when to say no. Here are a few ways to establish these boundaries:

- Define precise work hours and stick to them. Avoid the

temptation to check emails or complete tasks outside of these hours.
- Communicate your boundaries to colleagues, friends, and family. Let them know when you're available and when you're focusing on self-care or family time.
- Schedule breaks throughout your day for short walks, meditation, or simply to step away from your desk. These pauses can significantly reduce stress levels.

Tools for Mastering Time Management

In our digital age, numerous tools and techniques can help streamline our schedules and reduce stress. Here are a few worth considering:

- Digital Planners and Calendars: Apps like Google Calendar or Todoist allow you to organize your tasks and appointments efficiently, with reminders to keep you on track.
- Time Blocking: Allocate specific blocks of time to different tasks or activities. This method helps minimize multitasking, which can be a significant source of stress.
- The Pomodoro Technique: Work for 25 minutes, then take a 5-minute break. This technique can help maintain focus and prevent burnout.

Utilizing these tools can create a more manageable, less stressful daily routine supporting our gut health.

In closing, the relationship between time management and gut health is intricate, yet understanding it is crucial for our well-being. By recognizing the impact of stress on our digestive system, prioritizing tasks, setting boundaries, and employing practical tools to manage our time more efficiently, we can foster a lifestyle that supports our productivity and health. This holistic approach to wellness ensures that we're surviving our days and thriving with a resilient gut to match a balanced life.

As we move forward, let's remember the importance of nurturing our bodies and time, creating space for the things that truly matter.

MAKE A DIFFERENCE WITH YOUR REVIEW

Unlock the Power of Generosity

"Kindness is a language which the deaf can hear and the blind can see."

— MARK TWAIN

Did you know that people who help others without expecting anything in return often lead more joyful and successful lives? Well, if there's a chance to spread a little more joy in the world, I'm all in. And I have a small favor to ask you...

Would you be willing to help someone you've never met, without any recognition for your act of kindness?

Who might this person be, you wonder? They're a lot like you. Perhaps someone who's on the early part of a journey you've already navigated. Someone eager to make positive changes, searching for guidance, but unsure where to start.

Our mission with "Gut Health Unlocked" has always been to make the secrets to better gut health known to everyone. But to truly fulfill that mission, we need to reach as many people as possible.

This is where your generosity becomes invaluable. It turns out, reviews really do help others decide whether a book is right for them. So here's my request on behalf of a future reader you haven't met yet:

Could you spare a moment to help that reader by leaving a review for this book?

It doesn't cost a thing, takes barely a minute, but your words could be the nudge that someone else needs to start their journey toward better health. Your review might be the key that unlocks a world of difference for:

- Another family seeking ways to feel better together.
- A friend you haven't met yet who's looking for a sign to take the first step.
- Someone who's been feeling stuck and is in desperate need of inspiration.
- Or even a stranger who will finally find the guidance they've been searching for.

To share your thoughts and make a lasting impact, just:

Leave a review by scanning the QR code below:

If the thought of helping someone out there warms your heart, then you're exactly who I hoped to reach with this book. Welcome to our community. You're one of us now.

I'm thrilled at the opportunity to guide you to achieve remarkable gut health more smoothly and effectively than you ever imagined. The insights, stories, and strategies ahead are sure to enrich your journey.

With all my gratitude,

- Denise Smith Marsh

PS - Remember, sharing valuable insights makes you invaluable to others. If you believe "Gut Health Unlocked" can help someone you know, why not spread the kindness and recommend it? After all, happiness shared is happiness doubled.

NOURISHING THE FOUNDATION - HYDRATION AND ROUTINE FOR OPTIMAL GUT HEALTH

I magine a stream flowing gently through a dense, vibrant forest. This stream is the lifeblood of the forest, carrying vital nutrients, supporting lush vegetation, and sustaining the wildlife that calls it home. Now, picture your body as that forest and water as the stream. Just as the stream nourishes the forest, water nourishes your body, playing a pivotal role in every aspect of your health, especially your digestive system.

6.1 THE ROLE OF HYDRATION: WATER'S IMPACT ON DIGESTION

Water is critical to the digestive process, serving multiple roles that ensure everything runs smoothly. It breaks down food, allowing nutrients to be absorbed more easily. Water also helps dissolve vitamins, minerals, and other nutrients from food, facilitating their absorption into the bloodstream. It keeps the intestines smooth and flexible, aiding in the smooth passage of waste.

- **Lubricates the Intestines:** Imagine trying to slide down a dry water slide. It's not very fun, right? With adequate hydration, our intestines can move waste easily.
- **Facilitates Nutrient Absorption:** Water acts like a conveyor belt for nutrients, ensuring they reach their destination efficiently.
- **Aids in Digestion:** It's the first step in breaking down food, ensuring our body can access the nutrients it needs.

Signs of Dehydration

Recognizing the early signs of dehydration can prevent a cascade of digestive discomforts. Keep an eye out for:

- Thirst is the most obvious sign. If you feel thirsty, you're already on your way to dehydration.
- Urine color offers clues; dark yellow signifies a need for more fluids.
- Headaches and dizziness can also indicate dehydration, as can dry mouth and lips.
- Feeling unusually tired or lethargic during the day.

Daily Hydration Goals

How much water should you drink a day? The "8x8" rule (eight 8-ounce glasses) is easy to remember but doesn't fit everyone. Climate, activity level, and overall health play into your personal hydration needs. Start with:

- As a baseline, at least 64 ounces (about 1.9 liters) of water daily.
- Add 12-16 ounces before and after moderate exercise.
- Adjust based on the weather, increasing intake on hot or dry days.

Hydrating Foods

Incorporating water-rich foods into your diet is an enjoyable way to boost hydration. These foods can be especially beneficial in keeping you hydrated:

- Cucumbers and lettuce boast over 95% water content, making them top choices for hydration.
- Watermelon and strawberries satisfy a sweet tooth and are packed with water.
- Soups and broths, especially when loaded with vegetables, offer a comforting way to increase fluid intake.

Incorporate these into your daily meals by:

- Start your day with a smoothie made from watermelon, strawberries, and a splash of coconut water.
- Snack on cucumber slices or cherry tomatoes instead of less hydrating options.
- Add a side salad to your lunch and dinner.
- Opt for soups as part of your meals, especially in cooler weather.

Hydration is a cornerstone of good health, impacting our digestive system's efficiency. By recognizing the signs of dehydration, setting personal hydration goals, and including water-rich foods in our diet, we can support our digestive health while enjoying nature's variety and flavors. Remember, drinking water isn't just about quenching thirst; it's about nurturing our body's entire ecosystem, ensuring every process, especially digestion, has what it needs to function at its best.

6.2 HERBAL REMEDIES AND SUPPLEMENTS: WHAT WORKS?

Navigating the vast sea of herbal remedies and supplements can feel overwhelming in the quest for optimal gut health. Yet, amidst this complexity, certain herbs have emerged, backed by scientific evidence, as effective allies for our digestive system. In this section, we'll explore these herbs, understand how to select quality supplements, discuss the potential for interactions, and emphasize a tailored approach to supplementation.

Evidence-Based Herbal Remedies

Two standout herbs for gut health are ginger and peppermint. Both have a long history of traditional use, supported by contemporary research, for their digestive benefits:

- Ginger: Known for its warming properties, ginger can soothe an upset stomach, reduce nausea, and ease digestion. It accelerates gastric emptying and stimulates the digestive tract, making it less likely for discomfort and gas to build up. Ginger tea or supplements can be a simple yet effective way to incorporate this herb into your daily routine.

- Peppermint: With a refreshing and cooling effect, peppermint has been shown to relax the muscles of the digestive tract, which can help alleviate symptoms of IBS, such as cramping and bloating. Peppermint oil capsules, specifically enteric-coated ones designed to dissolve in the intestine, not the stomach, are particularly effective.

When incorporating these herbs into your regimen, starting with small doses and observing how your body responds is advisable. This cautious approach ensures you reap the benefits without overwhelming your system.

Choosing Quality Supplements

The supplement market is vast, and not all products are created equal. To ensure you're selecting high-quality supplements and herbs, here are some key points to consider:

- Third-Party Testing: Look for products independently tested and verified by third-party organizations. This testing can ensure the purity and potency of the supplement.
- Certification Marks: Certifications from organizations like the USP (United States Pharmacopeia) or NSF International indicate that the supplement meets strict quality and safety standards.
- Transparent Labeling: Choose supplements that clearly label the ingredients, including the specific strains of probiotics or the part of the herb used. This transparency is crucial for understanding what you're taking and its intended benefits.

Reviewing these criteria before adding any supplement to your routine can guide you toward safer, more effective options.

Potential Interactions

While herbal remedies and supplements offer numerous benefits, they're not without risks. One of the main concerns is the potential for interactions with medications. For example:

- Ginger: While beneficial for digestion, ginger can thin the blood, posing risks for individuals on blood-thinning medications.
- Peppermint: Although effective for IBS, peppermint can interact with medications that reduce stomach acid, potentially leading to heartburn or indigestion.

Given these complexities, it's paramount to consult with a healthcare provider before introducing herbal remedies or supplements, especially if you're currently taking medication. This precaution ensures your approach to gut health is both safe and effective.

Personalized Approach

Every individual's gut health journey is unique and influenced by personal health history, existing conditions, and specific needs. Adopting a personalized approach to supplementation means considering these factors to tailor your regimen for optimal benefits:

- Assess Your Needs: Reflect on your specific digestive issues and health goals. Are you seeking relief from bloating, aiming to enhance nutrient absorption, or looking to support overall digestive health?
- Start Slow: Introduce one supplement at a time and monitor your body's response. This method allows you to identify what works and adjust as needed.
- Continual Evaluation: Your body's needs can change over time. Regularly assess the effectiveness of your supplements and be willing to make adjustments in response to shifts in your health or goals.

This tailored strategy maximizes the benefits of herbal remedies and supplements and respects the individuality of your digestive system, ensuring a path to gut health that is as unique as you are.

Navigating the landscape of herbal remedies and supplements for gut health can be manageable. You can effectively support your digestive well-being by grounding your choices in evidence, prioritizing quality, being mindful of interactions, and adopting a personalized approach. Remember, the goal is to add more supplements to your diet and strategically enhance your gut health with well-chosen aids that harmonize with your body's needs.

6.3 THE POWER OF ROUTINE: STRUCTURING YOUR DAY FOR GUT HEALTH

Establishing a daily routine is akin to laying down a map of your body's internal processes. When you follow a consistent schedule, your digestive system learns to anticipate and prepare for meals, sleep, and stress management, leading to a smoother journey from waking up to closing your eyes at night. This predictability is crucial for reducing stress levels and enhancing digestive regularity, creating a harmonious environment for your gut health to thrive.

Crafting a Gut-Healthy Routine

To support your gut health effectively, consider weaving these practices into the fabric of your daily life:

- Meal Timing: Regularity in meal times trains your digestive system to kickstart the necessary processes for digestion and nutrient absorption at specific moments throughout the day. Aim to eat your meals around the same time daily, giving your body a clear signal of when to expect nourishment.
- Exercise: Integrating physical activity into your routine benefits your muscles and heart, as well as your gut. A brisk morning walk or a gentle yoga session can invigorate your digestive system, encouraging healthy bowel movements and enhancing the overall function of your gut. The key is consistency; even short bouts of activity can be profoundly beneficial when done regularly.
- Stress-Reduction Practices: It is vital to allocate time for activities that lower stress. Whether it's a few minutes of deep breathing, journaling, or engaging in a hobby, dedicating specific times for these activities can help manage stress levels and prevent the adverse effects of cortisol on your gut.

Incorporating these elements into your daily routine might

require some adjustments initially, but over time, they become second nature, providing a solid foundation for your gut health.

Flexibility Within Routine

While consistency is beneficial, life is inherently unpredictable. Flexibility within your routine allows you to adapt to unexpected changes without disrupting your gut health. Here's how you can maintain balance:

- Have a Plan B for Meals: If you're unable to eat at your usual time, having healthy snacks on hand can prevent long gaps between meals, keeping your digestion on track.
- Adaptable Exercise Options: If your usual workout isn't feasible, know some quick, at-home alternatives or stretches to keep the momentum without stressing about missing a session.
- Stress Management Tools: Equip yourself with various stress-relief techniques to choose the most practical option for any situation, whether it's a two-minute meditation session or simply stepping outside for a breath of fresh air.

This approach ensures your routine supports your gut health, even when life throws curveballs.

Routine and Sleep

The crown jewel of a gut-healthy routine is a well-structured nighttime ritual that paves the way for restorative sleep. Sleep is when the body repairs itself, and for the gut, this is used to process nutrients, regenerate cells, and balance microbiota. Here's how to create a sleep-promoting routine:

- Wind Down Before Bed: Slow down your activities and dim the lights at least an hour before your intended sleep time. This signals your body that it's time to shift into rest mode.
- Limit Late-Night Eating: Eating close to bedtime can lead to discomfort and disrupt your sleep. Try to have your last meal at least 2-3 hours before you sleep, allowing ample time for digestion.
- Prepare Your Sleep Environment: Make your bedroom a sleep sanctuary. A comfortable mattress, supportive pillows, and a cool temperature can significantly enhance the quality of your rest.
- Consistent Sleep Schedule: Going to bed and waking up at the same times each day, even on weekends, reinforces your body's sleep-wake cycle, improving sleep quality and supporting your gut health.

Nurture your body with a consistent, adaptable routine that prioritizes meal timing, exercise, stress reduction, and sleep to create an environment where your gut can function optimally. This doesn't just support your digestive system; it enhances your overall well-being, proving that sometimes, the simplest practices can have the most profound impact on our health.

6.4 HEALING THE GUT-BRAIN AXIS: A MINDFUL APPROACH

The connection between our gut and brain is more profound than many might realize. This intricate relationship, known as the gut-brain axis, is a two-way communication highway that affects how we think and feel and how well our digestive systems function. This axis underscores the importance of a balanced mind in maintaining a healthy gut and vice versa.

Gaining Insight into the Gut-Brain Axis

To appreciate the depth of the Gut-Brain connection, it's crucial to understand that the gut is often called the "second brain." This nickname stems from the vast network of neurons lining the gastrointestinal tract, which plays a crucial role in our emotions and physical health. The gut produces a significant amount of serotonin, a neurotransmitter that regulates mood, suggesting a direct link between digestive health and emotional well-being.

Mindfulness Practices for the Axis

To nurture this connection, incorporating mindfulness practices can be significantly beneficial. Here are a few focused approaches:

- Focused Breathing: This technique involves paying close attention to the breath, noticing how it feels as you inhale and exhale. This practice can calm the mind and, by extension, soothe the gut, especially during times of stress.
- Visualization Techniques: Visualizing a serene and healthy digestive system can reinforce the connection between mind and body. Picture your gut as a calm river,

smoothly flowing and nourishing your body. This mental imagery can promote peace and well-being throughout the digestive tract.

Both practices quiet the mind and create a more harmonious environment for the gut.

The Role of Emotional Regulation

Emotions can have a tangible impact on gut health, with stress, anxiety, and depression often exacerbating digestive issues. Managing these emotions through mindfulness can lead to improved gut health by:

- Reducing stress-induced inflammation in the gut.
- Decreasing stress-related digestive upset, such as irritable bowel syndrome (IBS) symptoms.
- Enhancing the overall function of the digestive system.

Strategies for healthy emotional regulation include acknowledging feelings without judgment, engaging in activities that bring joy, and practicing self-compassion. By addressing our emotional health, we directly contribute to the well-being of our gut.

Integrating Mindfulness into Daily Life

Making mindfulness a regular part of your day can help sustain the health of the gut-brain axis. Consider these integrations:

- Journaling: Daily writing down thoughts and feelings can provide clarity and reduce stress. Reflecting on daily experiences and the emotions they evoke can help

healthily process feelings, mitigating their impact on the gut.
- Mindful Movement: Activities such as yoga or tai chi combine physical movement with conscious awareness, offering dual benefits for the gut-brain axis. These practices encourage a focus on bodily sensations and breath, which can alleviate stress and support digestive health.

Incorporating these mindfulness practices into your routine doesn't require a significant time commitment or drastic lifestyle changes. Even a few minutes a day can make a noticeable difference in how you feel mentally and physically.

6.5 ENVIRONMENTAL FACTORS: YOUR SURROUNDINGS AND YOUR GUT

In a world where urban landscapes increasingly dominate our surroundings, it's easy to overlook the profound impact of the environment on our gut health. Every aspect of our environment shapes the microbial community within us, from the air we breathe to the water we drink. This section will peel back the layers on how pollution and toxins affect our gut health, guide you on creating a more gut-friendly living space, and shed light on the gut-health benefits of reconnecting with nature. Additionally, we'll touch on the importance of being mindful of the products we consume and how they can influence our gut microbiome.

Impact of Environment on Gut Health

Our guts are sensitive ecosystems that respond to the slightest changes in our surroundings. Exposure to pollutants and toxins, unfortunately common in urban environments, can disrupt the delicate balance of our gut microbiome. For instance, air pollution particles, when ingested or inhaled, can lead to inflammation in the gut, altering the composition of our microbiota. Similarly, pesticides and chemicals in non-organic produce can harm beneficial gut bacteria, leading to dysbiosis—a microbial imbalance linked to various health issues.

Creating a Gut-Healthy Environment

To foster a living space that supports your gut health, consider these adjustments:

- Reduce Chemical Exposure: Opt for natural cleaning products or make your own from vinegar, baking soda, and essential oils. These alternatives are less likely to introduce harmful chemicals into your home, offering a safer environment for your gut to thrive.
- Improve Indoor Air Quality: Indoor plants can act as natural air purifiers, removing toxins from the air. Additionally, ensure proper ventilation in your home to reduce pollutant concentration. Consider using air purifiers in rooms where you spend the most time to minimize further exposure to airborne toxins.
- Water Filtration: Installing a high-quality water filter can reduce exposure to tap water contaminants, such as chlorine and heavy metals, safeguarding your gut health.

These steps can transform your home into a sanctuary that nurtures rather than challenges your gut microbiome.

Nature and Gut Health

Spending time in natural surroundings can revitalize gut health. The diverse microbiomes found in outdoor environments can enrich our own, boosting microbial diversity and associated with better gut health and a more robust immune system. Activities like gardening expose you to beneficial soil-based organisms while walking in the forest can reduce stress levels, indirectly supporting gut health.

To integrate the healing power of nature into your routine:

- Regular Outdoor Activities: Make time for outdoor exercise or walks in green spaces. Combining physical activity and exposure to diverse microbes can enhance your gut health.
- Gardening: If space allows, start a small garden. Gardening connects you with beneficial microbes and provides fresh, pesticide-free produce that's good for your gut.

Mindful Consumption

The choices we make about what to consume extend beyond food. Products from skincare to household cleaners can contain additives and preservatives that might disrupt our gut microbiome.

To practice mindful consumption:

- Read Labels: Familiarize yourself with the ingredients in your products. Look for items free from artificial preservatives, fragrances, and dyes that can irritate the gut.

- **Choose Organic When Possible:** Organic food and personal care products are less likely to contain harmful chemicals that can upset your gut health.
- **Sustainable Choices:** Opt for products with minimal packaging to reduce exposure to plastics and chemicals. Sustainable choices are not only better for the planet but can also benefit your gut health.

Incorporating these practices into your life doesn't just contribute to a healthier gut; it fosters a more mindful and sustainable way of living. By being conscious of our environment and the products we bring into our homes, we can create a space that supports our gut health and overall well-being.

6.6 INTERMITTENT FASTING AND GUT HEALTH

Exploring the realm of gut health reveals a fascinating connection between the timing of our meals and the well-being of our digestive system. This connection is illuminated through intermittent fasting, a method that challenges traditional eating patterns and opens a pathway to restore and rejuvenate gut health. The foundation of intermittent fasting lies in its ability to give our digestive tract a break, allowing for periods of rest that can lead to an array of benefits, including improved microbial diversity and enhanced repair processes within the gut lining.

Understanding the Science Behind Fasting and Gut Restoration

At its core, intermittent fasting involves alternating cycles of eating and fasting. This practice isn't about which foods to eat but when to eat them. The science supporting intermittent fasting and gut health is compelling, as it points to improved gut barrier function, which is crucial for preventing harmful substances from leaking into the body. Additionally, fasting periods stimulate autophagy, a cellular "clean-up" process that removes damaged cells and parts, making room for new, healthy cells. This process is particularly beneficial for the cells lining the gut, as it can help repair and maintain a strong, intact intestinal barrier.

Moreover, fasting has been shown to influence the composition of the gut microbiota, promoting an increase in beneficial bacteria linked to anti-inflammatory properties and improved digestive health. These changes can contribute to a more balanced gut microbiome, which is critical in nutrient absorption and immune function.

Steps to Safely Practice Intermittent Fasting

While the benefits of intermittent fasting can be significant, it's crucial to approach this practice with care to ensure it aligns with your individual health needs and goals. Here are some steps to consider:

- Consult with a Professional: Before changing your eating patterns, especially if you have existing health conditions, it's wise to consult with a healthcare provider or a nutritionist. They can offer guidance on whether intermittent fasting suits you and how to apply it safely.
- Start Gradually: If you're new to intermittent fasting, begin with shorter fasting periods and gradually increase the duration as your body adjusts. A popular starting point is the 16/8 method, where you fast for 16 hours and eat within an 8-hour window.

- Listen to Your Body: Pay attention to how you feel during fasting periods. If you experience lightheadedness, excessive hunger, or irritability, adjusting your fasting schedule or consulting with a professional may be necessary for further guidance.
- Stay Hydrated: Drinking plenty of water during fasting periods is vital to prevent dehydration. Herbal teas and black coffee are also typically allowed and can help make fasting periods more manageable.

Personalizing Your Fasting Schedule

The effectiveness of intermittent fasting can vary widely among individuals, influenced by lifestyle, metabolism, and personal health factors. Therefore, personalizing your fasting schedule is vital to finding a rhythm that supports your gut health without disrupting your daily life. Consider the following:

- Align Fasting with Your Lifestyle: Choose fasting periods that fit naturally with your daily routine. For instance, if you're not a morning eater, skipping breakfast and starting your eating window later might work best for you.
- Adjust Based on Experience: As you experiment with intermittent fasting, note how different schedules affect your energy levels, digestion, and overall well-being. Use this feedback to fine-tune your fasting pattern.
- Incorporate Nutrient-Dense Foods: During eating windows, focus on nourishing your body with foods rich in fiber, vitamins, and minerals to support gut health. This ensures that when you eat, you provide your gut with the nutrients it needs to thrive.

In essence, intermittent fasting offers a unique approach to supporting gut health, emphasizing the importance of when we eat as much as what we eat. By understanding the underlying science, practicing fasting safely, and tailoring the approach to fit individual needs, this method can become a valuable tool in nurturing digestive wellness. Through careful application and personalization, intermittent fasting can help pave the way for a healthier, more balanced gut, contributing to overall health and vitality.

6.7 DETOXIFICATION AND GUT HEALTH

The concept of detoxification has woven itself into the fabric of health and wellness conversations, often presenting as a necessary ritual to purge our bodies of toxins. However, the narrative surrounding detox practices is rife with myths that can lead to confusion and, in some cases, more harm than good. It's crucial to sift through these myths, understanding that our bodies, particularly our liver and kidneys, are inherently equipped for detoxification. The real focus should be supporting these natural processes through safe and effective practices that contribute to gut health.

Many detox diets and cleanses promise rapid results, suggesting they can flush toxins from your body and improve gut health overnight. Yet, these extreme approaches are unnecessary and can disrupt the delicate balance of your gut microbiome. Instead, a gentler approach, emphasizing foods and habits that naturally support detoxification and gut health, is far more beneficial.

Debunking Detox Myths

The first step in adopting a healthy approach to detoxification is debunking common myths:

- Myth: Specific diets and products are required to detoxify the body. Fact: Your body is already a proficient detox machine. The liver, kidneys, and even your gut work tirelessly to filter out toxins without the need for drastic diets or expensive supplements.
- Myth: Detoxing leads to dramatic health improvements. Fact: True and lasting health improvements come from consistent, balanced eating habits and lifestyle choices, not short-term detox diets.

Safe and Effective Detox Practices for the Gut

Focusing on practices that support your body's natural detoxification processes can inadvertently boost your gut health:

- Stay Hydrated: Water is essential for the liver and kidneys to function optimally in filtering out toxins. It also keeps the digestive system running smoothly, preventing constipation and promoting regularity.
- Eat a Diet Rich in Fiber: Fiber aids in eliminating waste and toxins through regular bowel movements. Fiber foods such as fruits, vegetables, and whole grains also support a healthy gut microbiome.
- Limit Processed Foods: Reducing the intake of processed foods decreases the exposure to artificial additives and chemicals, which can burden your detoxification system and disrupt gut health.

Supplements and Herbs That Aid in Detoxification

While no supplement can "detox" your body in the way that fad diets claim, certain supplements and herbs can support the body's natural detoxification pathways and contribute to a healthy gut:

- Milk Thistle: Known for its liver-protecting qualities, milk thistle can support the liver in its detoxification roles. The liver processes nutrients absorbed from the gut and filters out toxins from the blood, making milk thistle a beneficial supplement for overall digestive health.
- Dandelion Root: Traditionally used to support kidney function, dandelion root acts as a diuretic, helping the kidneys flush out waste products efficiently. Its prebiotic fiber also nourishes the gut microbiome.
- Probiotics: These beneficial bacteria can indirectly support detoxification by maintaining a healthy gut barrier, preventing toxins from leaking from the gut into the bloodstream.

When considering supplements or herbs, choosing high-quality products and consulting with a healthcare professional is paramount, especially if you have existing health conditions or are taking medications.

By pivoting away from the myths of detoxification and towards practices that support our body's built-in detox systems, we foster a healthier gut and embrace a more sustainable approach to wellness. This shift allows us to focus on what truly matters: nourishing our bodies with what they need to carry out their natural processes effectively.

As we wrap up this exploration of detoxification and gut health, remember that the key to a healthy gut lies not in extreme cleanses or restrictive diets but in nurturing our bodies with hydration, a balanced diet rich in fiber, and, where appropriate, supplements that support our natural detoxification pathways. This approach simplifies our health pursuit and aligns with our body's innate wisdom and capabilities. Moving forward, let's carry with us the understanding that supporting our body's natural processes with gentle, nourishing practices is a profound act of care, setting the stage for lasting health and vitality.

UNRAVELING COMMON GUT CHALLENGES

Imagine biting into a crisp apple, feeling the crunch, tasting the sweetness, and then, unexpectedly, your stomach bloats like a balloon, ready for takeoff. Not the kind of lift-off you were hoping for, right? Bloating, alongside other gut health challenges, can turn even the best days sour. This chapter peels back the layers of one such pervasive issue: persistent bloating. Through understanding its roots and exploring practical solutions, we aim to deflate the mystery and discomfort of bloating, transforming your approach to gut health from the ground up.

7.1 NAVIGATING PERSISTENT BLOATING: CAUSES AND SOLUTIONS

Identifying Causes

Bloating can feel like you're carrying a heavy, invisible burden that's not just uncomfortable but often downright painful. Several culprits could be behind this unwelcome sensation:

- Food Intolerances: Dairy, gluten, and certain fruits and vegetables can be bloating triggers for some. It's like attending a party where you don't get along with a few guests, leading to tension and discomfort.
- Imbalanced Gut Bacteria: The gut microbiome is like a bustling city. If the balance between residents gets out of whack, it can lead to traffic jams and chaos, manifesting as bloating.
- Eating Habits: Eating too quickly, not chewing thoroughly, or dining on the run can introduce excess air into your digestive system, puffing up your stomach like a balloon.

Dietary Adjustments

Tweaking what and how you eat can often provide relief:

- Limit High-FODMAP Foods: Foods high in FODMAPs can be challenging for some people to digest, leading to gas and bloating. Imagine these foods as party crashers, causing trouble in your digestive system. Cutting back on them might restore peace.
- Increase Hydration: Drinking enough water is like smoothing the roads in the bustling city of your gut, helping everything move more smoothly and preventing traffic jams that lead to bloating.

Lifestyle Changes

Sometimes, it's not just about what you eat but also how you live:

- Regular Exercise: Movement helps keep the traffic in Gut City flowing. A simple walk or gentle yoga can move gas through your system.
- Stress Reduction Techniques: Stress can tighten your digestive tract, causing bloating. Techniques like deep breathing or meditation can help relax these pathways, like easing a tight knot.

When to Seek Help

If your bloating feels more like a constant companion than an occasional visitor, it might be time to seek professional advice:

- Persistent Symptoms: If changes to your diet and lifestyle aren't helping, or if bloating is accompanied by symptoms like weight loss, severe pain, or changes in your bowel habits, it's crucial to get checked out.
- Finding the Right Specialist: A gastroenterologist or a dietitian specializing in gut health can offer tailored advice. They're like detectives, helping to pinpoint the cause of your bloating and providing solutions tailored to your body's needs.

DIY Bloating Diary

Try keeping a bloating diary for a few weeks to get a clearer picture of what might be causing your bloating. Note what you eat, your stress levels, exercise habits, and when bloating occurs. Over time, patterns may emerge, offering clues to the culprits behind your discomfort.

Pro Tips for Immediate Bloating Relief

While long-term solutions are essential, sometimes you need quick relief:

- Peppermint Oil Capsules: Known for their soothing properties on the digestive tract, they can offer temporary relief from bloating.
- Warm Lemon Water: Starting your day with this can help kickstart your digestion and reduce morning bloating.
- Ginger Tea: A warm cup can help soothe your digestive system and reduce bloating, acting like a calm breeze through Gut City.

Mindful Eating Exercise

Slow your eating with this simple exercise: For your next meal, try putting down your utensil between bites. Chew thoroughly, savoring the flavors and textures. This enhances your dining experience, helps reduce the amount of air you swallow, and gives your digestive system a smoother ride.

Persistent bloating can be a frustrating, often confusing challenge. By understanding its potential causes, making thoughtful adjustments to your diet and lifestyle, and knowing when to seek professional advice, you can find relief and improve your gut health. Remember, the goal is not just to treat symptoms but to foster a healthier, more harmonious digestive system that supports your overall well-being.

7.2 COMBATING CHRONIC CONSTIPATION: A NEW APPROACH

Constipation can often feel like you're stuck at a crossroads, waiting for traffic to clear. Many factors contribute to this condition, making it a familiar yet uncomfortable topic. Let's navigate through the dietary and lifestyle adjustments, along with natural remedies, to create smoother paths for those struggling with chronic constipation.

Unraveling the Causes

Constipation is not just a single-issue scenario; it's a complex interplay of dietary habits, lifestyle choices, and, sometimes, underlying medical conditions. Low fiber intake, inadequate hydration, lack of physical activity, and certain medications can all lead to constipation. It's as if various roadblocks have been set up along your digestive tract, slowing traffic to a crawl. Understanding these contributing factors is the first step in formulating a plan to alleviate constipation.

The Role of Fiber

Integrating soluble and insoluble fiber into your diet acts like adding more lanes to a congested highway. Soluble fiber, which absorbs water and forms a gel-like substance, helps soften stools, making them easier to pass. Sources include oats, apples, and beans. Insoluble fiber, on the other hand, adds bulk to stools and can help speed up the passage of food through the digestive system. Think of whole grains, nuts, and vegetables as your go-to.

A balanced intake of both types of fiber is like ensuring your digestive tract has both the flexibility and the capacity to handle what comes its way. Gradually increase your fiber intake to give your body time to adjust, and aim for about 25 to 30 grams of fiber per day for optimal results.

Hydration and Exercise: Twin Pillars of Regularity

Pairing adequate hydration with regular exercise can significantly impact maintaining bowel regularity. Water keeps the digestive system flowing, ensuring fiber can do its job effectively. Aim for at least eight glasses of water daily, more if you're active or it's hot outside.

Meanwhile, exercise gets everything moving, not just your muscles but your bowels. Engaging in moderate activity, such as walking, swimming, or cycling, for at least 30 minutes most days a week can help stimulate intestinal contractions, moving stools through more smoothly.

Embracing Natural Remedies

Sometimes, our bodies need a gentle nudge to get back on track. Several natural remedies and supplements can safely aid in relieving constipation:

- Probiotics: These beneficial bacteria can help balance the gut microbiome, potentially easing constipation. They enhance gut motility, helping regulate traffic flow in your digestive tract. Yogurt, kefir, and fermented foods are excellent food sources, while supplements can also be an option.
- Magnesium: This mineral can have a natural laxative effect, drawing water into the intestines and making stools easier to pass. Foods rich in magnesium include spinach, almonds, and whole grains. Supplements are available but start with a low dose to see how your body responds.
- Herbal Teas: Certain herbal teas, such as senna or dandelion, can gently stimulate bowel movements. However, it is important to use these teas cautiously, as overuse can lead to dependency.

These natural approaches offer a gentler alternative to over-the-counter laxatives, which should only be used as a last resort and under the guidance of a healthcare professional.

A multifaceted plan that includes dietary changes, lifestyle adjustments, and natural remedies can often lead to relief from chronic constipation. Remember, what works for one person may not work for another, so it's important to listen to your body and adjust your approach as needed. This personalized strategy ensures your digestive tract is not just moving but thriving, setting the stage for improved gut health and overall well-being.

7.3 DEALING WITH DIARRHEA: DIETARY AND LIFESTYLE CHANGES

Diarrhea, while often a topic skirted around in polite conversation, is a common issue that can significantly disrupt daily life. It can stem from various sources, ranging from dietary choices to stress levels, and understanding how to mitigate its effects can restore both gut balance and peace of mind. This section aims to navigate the turbulent waters of managing diarrhea through careful diet and lifestyle modifications.

Identifying Triggers

Pinpointing the exact causes of diarrhea can feel like solving a complex puzzle, especially when multiple factors could be at play. Start by observing your dietary habits closely. Foods that are high in fats, artificial sweeteners, or even dairy products for those with lactose intolerance can often precipitate diarrhea. Similarly, caffeine and alcohol have a laxative effect on some individuals, speeding up digestion too much for comfort.

On another front, stress and anxiety can also play significant roles in triggering diarrhea. The gut-brain axis, a communication network linking the emotional and cognitive centers of the brain with peripheral intestinal functions, can become activated during stress, leading to gastrointestinal symptoms, including diarrhea.

BRAT Diet and Beyond

When diarrhea strikes, turning to the BRAT diet—bananas, rice, applesauce, and toast—can be a helpful initial step. These foods are bland, easy on the stomach, and help bind stools, making them firmer. Here's a closer look at how each component helps:

- Bananas: Rich in potassium, they help replenish electrolytes lost during diarrhea episodes.
- Rice: Its simplicity and lack of fiber make it easy to digest, reducing the strain on a troubled digestive system.
- Applesauce: Provides pectin, a soluble fiber that can help absorb excess liquid in the intestines.
- Toast: Slightly charred bread dries the stools and provides needed energy without overstimulating the gut.

Expanding beyond the BRAT diet and incorporating other gentle foods over time aids in recovery. Boiled potatoes, steamed chicken, or clear broths can also provide nourishment without aggravating the digestive tract. Remember, the reintroduction of regular foods should be gradual to avoid overwhelming a sensitive system.

Probiotic Support

Probiotics, the beneficial bacteria in our gut, play a crucial role in maintaining digestive health and can be especially helpful in managing diarrhea. Certain strains of probiotics, such as Lactobacillus rhamnosus GG and Saccharomyces boulardii, have shown effectiveness in reducing the duration and intensity of diarrhea episodes, particularly those caused by antibiotics or infections.

Incorporating probiotics into your diet doesn't have to be complicated. Yogurt with live cultures, kefir, and fermented foods such as sauerkraut or kimchi introduce these helpful bacteria into your gut. Probiotic supplements can also be an option for more targeted support, offering specific strains in concentrated doses. If choosing a supplement, look for products with research supporting their efficacy for diarrhea and consult a healthcare provider to ensure they fit your needs well.

Stress Management Techniques

Since stress can directly impact gut function and contribute to episodes of diarrhea, finding effective ways to manage stress is vital. Simple practices can significantly affect how your body responds to stressors, reducing the frequency and severity of diarrhea. Here are a few techniques to consider:

- Mindfulness Meditation: Spending a few minutes each day in meditation can lower stress levels and, by extension, calm the digestive tract. Focus on your breath and allow thoughts to pass without engaging them, fostering a sense of peace and stillness.
- Regular Exercise: Physical activity releases endorphins, which are natural mood elevators that can reduce stress. Walking, swimming, or yoga support overall health and moderate the body's stress response.
- Adequate Sleep: Ensuring you get enough restorative sleep is vital for stress management. Establish a calming bedtime routine and aim for 7-9 hours of sleep per night to help your body and mind recover from the day's stresses.

- Time Management: Organizing your day to avoid last-minute rushes can decrease stress levels. Use planners or digital apps to schedule tasks, including regular breathing breaks and regrouping.

You can significantly improve your gut health and overall well-being by addressing the dietary and lifestyle factors that often contribute to diarrhea. From carefully selecting foods that support digestion to managing stress and incorporating probiotics, these strategies offer a roadmap to a more comfortable and balanced digestive function.

7.4 TACKLING FOOD INTOLERANCES HEAD-ON

Understanding and managing food intolerances is vital in the realm of gut health. Unlike food allergies, which can cause immediate and potentially life-threatening reactions, food intolerances primarily affect the digestive system, leading to discomfort and sometimes severe symptoms. The distinction lies in the severity and the body's response; intolerances involve the digestive system's failure to properly break down certain foods, while allergies trigger the immune system.

Recognizing Food Intolerances

Food intolerances can be sneaky, with symptoms ranging from gas and bloating to diarrhea, constipation, and even fatigue, making them challenging to pinpoint. The key to detection lies in observing your body's reactions to specific foods. If certain items consistently lead to digestive distress, they might be the culprits. Common triggers include lactose in dairy products, gluten in wheat, barley, and rye, and certain types of carbohydrates that ferment in the gut.

Elimination Diet Guidance

An elimination diet is a powerful tool for identifying food intolerances. The process involves removing suspected foods from your diet for a period, then gradually reintroducing them to observe potential reactions. Here's a step-by-step guide to conducting an effective elimination diet:

- Step 1: Planning - List foods you suspect may be causing issues. Common culprits include dairy, gluten, soy, eggs, and nuts.
- Step 2: Elimination—For 3-4 weeks, remove these foods from your diet altogether. It's crucial during this phase to read labels carefully and avoid hidden sources of these foods.
- Step 3: Monitoring—During the elimination phase, Keep a detailed food diary, noting what you eat and any symptoms you experience.
- Step 4: Reintroduction - After the elimination period, reintroduce one food group every three days. Note any changes in symptoms in your food diary.

This systematic approach can help isolate specific food intolerances, clarifying which foods your body can comfortably digest and which cannot.

Reintroducing Foods

The reintroduction phase is critical in the elimination diet. It requires patience and attention to detail. To ensure accuracy:

- Introduce Only One Food at a Time: This helps isolate reactions to specific foods.
- Start with Small Amounts: Begin by consuming a small portion of the reintroduced food, gradually increasing it over the three days unless symptoms occur.
- Record Everything: Continue using your food diary to track what you eat and any symptoms. This detailed record is invaluable for identifying intolerances.

Living with Intolerances

Discovering you have food intolerances doesn't mean you have to live in fear of food. With some adjustments, you can enjoy a diverse and satisfying diet:

- Learn to Read Labels: Understanding food labels is crucial to avoid ingesting your trigger foods inadvertently.
- Find Substitutes: For nearly every food intolerance, a substitute can help you enjoy your favorite dishes. Dairy-free milk, gluten-free grains, and egg replacers are just a few examples.
- Cook at Home: Preparing meals gives you complete control over the ingredients, ensuring you avoid those you're intolerant to.
- Communicate When Dining Out: When dining out, don't hesitate to ask about the ingredients in dishes and clearly

communicate your dietary restrictions. Most restaurants are accustomed to accommodating such requests.

The landscape of eating and enjoying food changes for those with food intolerances. However, it doesn't have to be limiting. With the proper knowledge and strategies, you can successfully navigate your dietary needs, ensuring your gut health and overall well-being remain in harmony.

7.5 OVERCOMING THE ANXIETY OF EATING OUT WITH GUT ISSUES

Navigating dining out's social and culinary landscape can often feel daunting for those managing gut health issues. The unpredictability of menu options, the challenge of communicating dietary needs, and the fear of unexpected gut reactions can make restaurant meals seem like a minefield. However, with some forethought and strategy, you can enjoy eating out, turning it into a positive experience rather than a source of stress.

Preparation is Key

Before stepping out, homework can go a long way in ensuring a smooth dining experience. Start by choosing restaurants known for accommodating dietary restrictions or having a diverse menu that includes cleaner, more straightforward dishes. Many establishments now offer their menus online, providing the perfect opportunity to scout potential meals that align with your dietary needs. If the menu leaves you with questions, don't hesitate to call the restaurant beforehand. A brief conversation can clarify whether they can cater to your needs, giving you peace of mind before you arrive.

Communicating Needs

Once at the restaurant, clear communication is your best tool for a safe and satisfying meal. Wait staff are your allies in this endeavor, and most are more than willing to assist if you approach them with specific and polite requests. Here are some practical ways to convey your dietary restrictions:

- Be concise but clear about your needs, avoiding overly technical language that might confuse.
- Mention that your restrictions are health-related, often prompting staff to take extra care.
- Ask for recommendations within your dietary framework, showing openness to suggestions.

Choosing Wisely

Making smart choices from the menu requires a balance between caution and enjoyment. Here's how to navigate your options:

- Opt for dishes with simple, whole-food ingredients. These are typically easier on the gut and minimize the risk of hidden triggers.
- Inquire about preparation methods. Grilled, baked, or steamed options are generally safer bets than fried or creamy dishes.
- Consider side dishes or appetizers as main courses if they offer safer ingredients for your dietary needs.

Mindful Eating Practices

Eating mindfully is especially crucial when dining out. The novel environment and the social aspect of eating in a restaurant can easily lead to rushed eating, which could be better for digestion. Here are a few mindful eating tips to help you enjoy your meal and minimize the risk of discomfort:

- Take small bites, chew thoroughly, and put your utensil down between bites to slow down the pace of eating.
- Stay present. Engage your senses fully with each bite, appreciating your food's flavors, textures, and aromas.
- Listen to your body's signals. Stop eating when you feel satisfied but not overly full, as overeating can exacerbate gut issues.

By adopting these approaches, dining out becomes less about navigating a dietary minefield and more about enjoying the pleasures of good food and company, all while keeping your gut health in check.

In wrapping up, it's clear that with thoughtful preparation, clear communication, wise menu choices, and mindful eating practices, the experience of dining out can remain a delightful part of life, even for those of us aware of our gut health. These strategies alleviate the anxiety associated with eating out and empower us to control our dietary needs without sacrificing the joy of a meal shared with friends or family. As we move forward, let's carry with us the understanding that our dietary restrictions do not define our social lives but offer us an opportunity to navigate the culinary world more thoughtfully and intentionally.

GUT HEALTH AND WEIGHT MANAGEMENT

Imagine stepping onto a scale, not with trepidation, but with a sense of understanding and control over the number you see. This isn't about quick fixes or restrictive diets that leave you feeling deprived. It's about tuning into the world within your gut, where trillions of bacteria reside, each playing a crucial role in your overall health, including your weight. The connection between these microscopic inhabitants and our waistlines is profound, shedding light on why some people struggle with weight despite their best efforts. In contrast, others seem to maintain a healthy weight effortlessly.

The gut microbiome, our inner ecosystem, is a bustling metropolis of bacteria, each species with its own role in digesting food, regulating hormones, and even controlling hunger and satiety signals. It's time to explore how adjusting this internal community can be a game-changer in managing weight. By understanding the microbiome-weight connection, identifying prebiotic and probiotic strains that aid in weight management, and making targeted adjustments to our microbiome, we can unlock a new level of control over our health and weight.

8.1 THE MICROBIOME-WEIGHT CONNECTION

The link between gut bacteria and weight is a fascinating research area gaining traction. Studies have shown that the composition of our gut microbiome can influence fat storage, how we balance blood sugar levels, and even how we respond to hormones that make us feel hungry or full. This means that the types of bacteria in our gut can play a pivotal role in determining our weight.

For instance, certain gut bacteria can extract more calories from our food, contributing to weight gain. Others impact how we store fat, influencing whether we're more likely to put on pounds. Moreover, some microbial strains affect how we regulate blood sugar, impacting hunger and energy levels throughout the day.

Adjusting Your Microbiome for Weight Loss

Adjusting the balance of our gut microbiome for weight loss isn't about drastic dietary overhauls. It's about making strategic tweaks that encourage the growth of beneficial bacteria. Here's how:

- Fiber-Rich Foods: Prebiotic fibers in foods like bananas, asparagus, and onions nourish good bacteria, helping them thrive.
- Fermented Foods: Incorporating yogurt, kefir, sauerkraut, and kombucha introduces probiotics, beneficial bacteria that can enhance gut health and support weight management.

- Diverse Diet: Eating a wide variety of foods can promote a diverse microbiome, which is linked to better weight control and overall health.

Prebiotic and Probiotic Strains That Aid in Weight Management

Not all bacteria are created equal when it comes to weight management. Specific strains have been identified for their potential benefits:

- Lactobacillus rhamnosus: Some studies have shown that this probiotic strain aids in weight loss and fat loss, making it a star player in the weight management lineup.
- Bifidobacterium lactis: Known for improving gut health, this strain may also help regulate body mass and reduce waist circumference.
- Prebiotic fibers: While not a bacterial strain, prebiotic fibers such as inulin and oligofructose nourish beneficial bacteria, promoting a balanced microbiome that supports healthy weight.

Incorporating these specific strains through diet or supplements can be a strategic move in managing weight. However, it's essential to approach supplementation with care, opting for high-quality products and consulting with a healthcare professional, especially if you have existing health conditions.

The journey to understanding and adjusting our microbiome for weight management is a testament to the power of our inner ecosystem. By fostering a gut environment that supports health and balance, we can unlock new pathways to managing weight and breaking free from the cycle of dieting and frustration. This approach isn't just about the numbers on a scale; it's about nurturing our bodies from the inside out, creating a foundation of health that supports our goals naturally and sustainably.

8.2 DIETARY STRATEGIES FOR A BALANCED MICROBIOME

Navigating the landscape of gut health necessitates a nuanced understanding of what fuels the bustling city of microbes within us. Daily food choices act as the infrastructure, either supporting a thriving metropolis of beneficial bacteria or leading to an imbalanced ecosystem prone to disruptions. To cultivate a microbiome that backs our weight management efforts and overall well-being, we must be mindful of the foods we introduce into this delicate environment.

Foods to Embrace and Avoid for a Healthy Gut

Our dietary habits play a pivotal role in shaping the composition and functionality of our gut microbiome. To foster a beneficial bacterial community, consider the following guidelines:

Foods to Embrace

- Diverse Plant-Based Foods: A varied diet rich in vegetables, fruits, legumes, and whole grains offers a spectrum of fibers and phytonutrients that feed good bacteria.
- Lean Proteins: Incorporating lean protein sources, such as poultry, fish, and plant-based alternatives, can support gut health without overwhelming it with hard-to-digest fats.
- Healthy Fats: Avocados, nuts, seeds, and olive oil provide

essential fatty acids that encourage the growth of health-promoting gut bacteria.

Foods to Avoid

- Processed and Sugary Foods: These can promote the growth of harmful bacteria and yeast, leading to an imbalanced microbiome.
- Artificial Sweeteners: Some studies suggest that artificial sweeteners may negatively affect gut bacteria and lead to glucose intolerance.
- Red and Processed Meats: High consumption of these foods has been linked to adverse changes in gut microbiota and an increased risk of certain diseases.

By curating our plates and emphasizing whole, unprocessed foods, we create an environment where beneficial microbes can flourish, supporting our gut health and weight management efforts.

Creating a Microbiome-Friendly Meal Plan

Designing a meal plan that nurtures our gut microbiota involves more than just choosing the right foods; it's about creating harmony and balance in our daily intake. Here are steps to craft a microbiome-friendly meal plan:

1. Start with Variety: Each meal should incorporate a rainbow of plant-based foods, ensuring a broad intake of fibers and nutrients to feed diverse bacterial species.
2. Incorporate Fermented Foods: Daily servings of yogurt,

kefir, sauerkraut, or kimchi introduce live probiotics into the gut, bolstering microbial diversity.
3. Balance Macronutrients: Ensuring each meal has a healthy balance of carbohydrates, proteins, and fats supports sustained energy levels and gut health.
4. Plan for Prebiotics: To fuel beneficial bacteria, regularly include prebiotic-rich foods like garlic, onions, bananas, and asparagus.
5. Stay Hydrated: Adequate water intake is crucial for maintaining a healthy mucus layer in the gut, where many beneficial bacteria reside.

This approach supports the microbiome and aligns with broader health goals, crafting a path toward sustainable well-being.

Timing Your Meals for Optimal Gut Health

The timing of our meals can influence the gut microbiome's composition and function, impacting everything from digestion to nutrient absorption. Here's how to optimize meal timing for gut health:

- Consistent Eating Schedule: Regular eating helps regulate the body's internal clock, supporting digestive processes and microbial rhythms.
- Mindful of Nighttime Eating: Limiting food intake hours before bed allows the gut to rest and repair, reducing the risk of indigestion and supporting a healthy circadian rhythm.
- Spacing Meals and Snacks: Allowing a few hours between meals and snacks gives the gut time to process food and can prevent overfeeding specific bacterial populations.

Adapting our eating habits to what we eat and when we eat can profoundly affect our gut microbiome, harmonizing our internal ecosystem with our body's natural rhythms. This synchronization supports digestive health and our broader metabolic and physiological processes, underscoring the intricate connection between our lifestyle choices and the microbial world within.

8.3 MINDFULNESS AND WEIGHT LOSS

Understanding the psychological layers that intertwine with our eating habits unlocks a new dimension in managing weight. Our mental state, emotions, and the environment significantly influence our food choices and eating behaviors, often in ways we might not fully realize. Incorporating mindfulness into our relationship with food invites a moment of pause, a breath between impulse and action, allowing us to make choices that align more closely with our health and weight goals.

The Psychological Aspects of Eating and Weight

Eating is more than just a physical act to satiate hunger; it's also an emotional and psychological experience. Stress, boredom, sadness, and even joy can drive us to seek comfort in food, leading to patterns that may not align with our health goals. The key is to recognize these emotional triggers and understand their role in our eating habits. This awareness can help us break free from the cycle of emotional eating and develop a healthier relationship with food.

Mindful Practices to Support Weight Management

Mindfulness, the practice of being fully present and engaged at the moment without judgment, can transform our eating and weight management approach. Here are some mindful practices to consider:

- Mindful Eating Exercises: Slow down and savor your food. Notice the colors, textures, and flavors. Chew slowly and put down your utensils between bites. This practice encourages you to enjoy your food more thoroughly, often leading to less eating.
- Body Scan Meditation: Before a meal, take a few moments to perform a quick body scan meditation. This helps you tune into your body's actual hunger signals and distinguish them from emotional or stress-induced eating urges.
- Breathing Techniques: Stress can lead to impulsive eating. When you feel overwhelmed, try a few deep breathing exercises to center yourself before making food choices.

Incorporating these practices into your daily routine can foster a more mindful, intentional approach to eating and support your weight management efforts.

Setting Realistic Goals and Celebrating Progress

Achieving lasting weight management is a gradual process that involves setting realistic, achievable goals. These goals should be specific, measurable, attainable, relevant, and time-bound (SMART). Here's how to approach goal-setting mindfully:

- Start Small: Focus on small, incremental changes you can build upon, like incorporating one extra serving of

vegetables into your daily diet or practicing mindful eating at one meal a day.
- Track Your Progress: Keep a journal of your food intake, mindful eating practices, and reflections on how you feel physically and emotionally. This record can help you identify patterns and celebrate your progress.
- Practice Self-Compassion: Be kind to yourself on this journey. Recognize that setbacks are part of the process and an opportunity for learning and growth.

Celebrating your progress, no matter how small, is crucial. Each step forward is a victory, contributing to a more significant transformation. Acknowledging your efforts reinforces positive behavior and motivates you to continue.

In weaving mindfulness into our approach to eating and weight, we tap into a powerful tool that aligns our actions with our intentions. This practice supports weight management and enhances our overall well-being, creating a harmonious relationship with food, our bodies, and our minds.

As we wrap up this mindfulness and weight loss exploration, we're reminded of the intricate dance between our physical and emotional selves. The mindful practices we've discussed offer a pathway to navigate this terrain gracefully, making choices that nourish our bodies and spirits. This journey isn't just about the food on our plates or the numbers on a scale; it's about cultivating awareness, kindness, and a deeper connection to ourselves. As we move forward, let us carry this mindfulness with us, allowing it to illuminate our path toward health, balance, and well-being.

DEMYSTIFYING THE GUT HEALTH CONUNDRUMS

Imagine standing in front of a vast, intricate network of pathways, each leading to different aspects of health and wellness. This network represents the gut, a complex system where the right balance can lead to harmony, and any imbalance may result in a cascade of health issues. In this chapter, we peel back the layers of common conundrums surrounding gut health, unraveling the mysteries with practical insights and actionable advice. Our focus is on understanding these complexities and navigating them easily, making informed decisions about our gut health.

9.1 DO PROBIOTICS WORK FOR EVERYONE? UNDERSTANDING THE VARIABILITY

The buzz around probiotics has grown louder over the years, promising to transform gut health and enhance overall well-being. Yet, a question lingers—do probiotics work the same magic for everyone?

Individual Responses

The human gut is as unique as a fingerprint, populated by many bacteria, viruses, and fungi that differ from person to person. These differences mean that what works for one individual may only sometimes work for another. Genetics, diet, lifestyle, and even previous antibiotic use can influence how one's body responds to probiotics. It's like planting the same seed in different soils; the growth depends on the soil's condition, not just the seed's potential.

Selecting the Right Strains

With shelves teeming with probiotic supplements, each boasting various strains, selecting the right one can feel overwhelming. The key lies in matching the probiotic strain to your specific health needs. For instance, Lactobacillus rhamnosus GG has been linked to reducing antibiotic-associated diarrhea, while Bifidobacterium lactis may help improve digestion. Consulting with a healthcare provider can shed light on which strains might be most beneficial based on your health history and goals.

Trial and Error

Finding the most effective probiotic often requires a trial-and-error approach. Start with one probiotic strain or a blend recommended for your concern and monitor your body's response. If you notice improvements, that's great! If not, it might be time to try a different strain or blend. Keeping a gut health journal can help track changes and pinpoint what works best for you during this process.

Alternative Sources

For those who find probiotic supplements have yet to hit the mark, turning to natural sources is the answer. Fermented foods like yogurt, kefir, sauerkraut, and kombucha are rich in probiotics. Incorporating these foods into your daily diet can bolster your gut flora naturally. Plus, they bring a wealth of nutrients and flavors to your meals, making gut health endeavors delicious and nutritious.

Visual Element: A chart comparing probiotic strains and their linked health benefits could help readers visualize which probiotics might suit their needs.

Textual Element: A checklist for monitoring changes while trying new probiotics or fermented foods, focusing on symptoms, overall well-being, and adverse reactions.

This exploration into the world of probiotics reveals the nuanced nature of gut health. While probiotics offer promising benefits, understanding individual variability, selecting suitable strains, and being open to trial and error pave the way to optimizing gut health. Fermented foods emerge as a tasty alternative and a cornerstone of a gut-friendly diet, offering a holistic approach to nurturing our microbiome.

9.2 CAN GUT HEALTH AFFECT MY MOOD AND ENERGY LEVELS?

The intricate dance between our gut and brain, known as the gut-brain axis, is a testament to the body's complexity. This dynamic connection underscores gut health's profound impact on our emotional and physical state, particularly our mood and energy levels.

Gut-Brain Axis

At the heart of this relationship is a two-way communication system that links our brain's emotional and cognitive centers with peripheral intestinal functions. This axis not only ensures the basic functioning of digestion but also plays a crucial role in our mental state. For instance, have you ever felt "butterflies" in your stomach when nervous? That's the gut-brain axis at work. This connection means that an imbalance in our gut can directly influence our mood, leading to feelings of anxiety or depression. Conversely, stress can impact our gut health, creating a cyclic effect.

Microbiome and Neurotransmitters

One of the most fascinating aspects of this relationship is the role of the gut microbiome in neurotransmitter production. Neurotransmitters are chemical messengers that play a significant role in mood regulation, including serotonin, often called the "happy chemical" for its role in promoting well-being and happiness. Astonishingly, up to 95% of serotonin is produced in the gut, not the brain, highlighting the gut's significant role in our emotional health. An imbalanced microbiome may produce insufficient serotonin and other neurotransmitters, affecting mood and energy levels.

Dietary Impacts

What we eat directly influences the composition of our gut microbiome, affecting our mood and energy. Diets high in processed foods, sugar, and saturated fats can contribute to dysbiosis, an imbalance in gut bacteria. This imbalance can reduce the production of neurotransmitters in the gut, contributing to mood disorders. On the other hand, a diet rich in whole foods, fibers, and fermented foods can promote a healthy microbiome, enhancing neurotransmitter production and, by extension, improving mood and energy levels.

- Fiber-Rich Foods: Foods high in fiber, such as fruits, vegetables, and whole grains, help feed beneficial gut bacteria, promoting their growth and activity.
- Fermented Foods: Foods like yogurt, kefir, sauerkraut, and kombucha introduce beneficial bacteria into the gut, contributing to a balanced microbiome.
- Omega-3 Fatty Acids: Found in fish, flaxseed, and walnuts, omega-3 fatty acids have been linked to reduced rates of depression, likely through their beneficial effects on the microbiome.

Holistic Management Strategies

Given the complexity of the gut-brain relationship, a holistic approach to managing gut health can improve mood and energy. This approach encompasses dietary and lifestyle modifications that reduce stress and improve sleep, which is integral to gut and mental health.

- Stress Management: Techniques such as yoga, meditation, and deep-breathing exercises can reduce stress and limit its impact on gut health and mood.
- Sleep Hygiene: Establishing a regular sleep schedule, reducing screen time before bed, and creating a calming bedtime routine can improve sleep quality and positively affect gut health and mood.

- Exercise: Regular physical activity can boost mood and energy levels by enhancing the growth of beneficial gut bacteria.

Incorporating these strategies into daily life can create a positive feedback loop. Improving gut health enhances mood and energy, which in turn motivates continued healthy habits. This holistic approach underscores the interconnectedness of our bodily systems, revealing the power of the gut to influence not only our physical health but also our mental well-being.

9.3 IS IT TOO LATE TO IMPROVE MY GUT HEALTH?

The passing years bring wisdom, experiences, and sometimes, a sense of resignation towards our health. However, when it comes to improving gut health, the clock hasn't run out, regardless of the number on your birthday cake. The human body remains a marvel of adaptability, and the gut is no exception. Our bodies respond positively to diet, lifestyle, and mindset changes as we age.

Age-Related Changes

As we age, our bodies undergo transformations that can affect every system, including the gut. These changes can lead to alterations in gut microbiota, digestive enzymes, and stomach acidity. While these shifts might sound daunting, they open up a dialogue about the importance of gut health and the possibility of positive intervention at any stage of life. It's not about turning back the clock but fine-tuning the body's current state to enhance well-being.

Success Stories

Countless individuals have rewritten their health narratives, proving it's always possible to start caring for your gut. Consider the case of a retired teacher who, after decades of digestive discomfort and fatigue, decided to take charge of her gut health. Through gradual dietary changes and the incorporation of gentle, gut-friendly exercises into her routine, she experienced remarkable improvements in digestion, energy levels, and even mental clarity. Her story, among others, serves as a beacon of hope, illustrating that positive changes are within reach, irrespective of age.

Step-by-Step Approach

Embarking on the path to better gut health doesn't require drastic measures. Instead, a gradual approach, rooted in consistency and patience, yields the most sustainable results. Here's how to begin:

- Dietary Changes: To support healthy digestion and gut flora, start by introducing more fiber-rich foods into your diet. Incorporate a variety of fruits, vegetables, whole grains, and legumes. Simultaneously, reduce your intake of processed foods, sugars, and unhealthy fats that can disrupt gut balance.
- Supplementation: Consider adding a probiotic supplement to your routine, especially if your diet lacks fermented foods. Probiotics can help replenish and maintain a healthy balance of gut bacteria. However, opt for supplements with strains proven to support gut health and consult a healthcare professional before starting any new supplement.

- Lifestyle Modifications: Increase your physical activity with options that you enjoy and are feasible for your lifestyle, such as walking, swimming, or yoga. Physical activity can stimulate digestion and reduce stress, a common contributor to gut health issues. Additionally, prioritize getting enough sleep and practice stress-reduction techniques like meditation or deep breathing exercises.
- Hydration: Ensure you're drinking enough water throughout the day. Proper hydration is crucial for digestion and can help prevent constipation, a common issue as we age.

Professional Support

While the journey to improved gut health can start with individual actions, seeking professional guidance ensures your efforts are tailored to your unique needs and conditions. A healthcare provider can offer personalized advice, help identify underlying issues, and recommend specific dietary changes or supplements. Additionally, a dietitian specializing in gut health can provide valuable insights into creating a diet plan that supports your gut health goals.

Recognizing the body's resilience and capacity for renewal debunks the notion that it's too late to improve gut health. With each tiny, consistent step, the gut can regain balance, enhancing overall health and vitality. Through a blend of dietary adjustments, lifestyle changes, and professional guidance, revitalizing your gut health is possible and a reality, regardless of age.

9.4 HOW CAN I TELL IF MY GUT HEALTH IS IMPROVING?

How do we recognize real progress in pursuing better gut health? After all, the signs of improvement can be subtle; sometimes, the body speaks in whispers rather than shouts. Here, we explore varied, practical ways to gauge the positive changes in your gut health, ensuring you can acknowledge and celebrate every step forward in this nuanced aspect of well-being.

Symptom Tracking

One of the most direct methods to observe the shifts in your gut health is by keeping a detailed symptom diary. This simple yet effective tool can help you connect the dots between your lifestyle choices and your digestive health. Here's how to go about it:

- Daily Entries: Make it a habit to jot down any gastrointestinal symptoms you experience daily. Include details such as the time of day, severity, and duration of symptoms like bloating, gas, discomfort, or irregular bowel movements.
- Dietary Notes: Alongside symptom tracking, note what you eat and drink. This parallel record helps identify foods that either trigger discomfort or promote well-being.
- Lifestyle Factors: Remember to document your stress levels, physical activity, and sleep quality. These can play significant roles in gut health and help you understand what contributes to your symptoms or lack thereof.

Over time, this diary will become a valuable resource, offering insights into patterns and trends that can guide further adjustments to your gut health strategies.

Biofeedback Tools

For those inclined towards more quantitative data, various biofeedback tools can better understand your gut health status. Here are a couple of options:

- Stool Analysis: At-home stool test kits have become more accessible and can provide information on aspects like bacterial diversity, the presence of specific beneficial or harmful bacteria, and markers of inflammation. While these tests should not replace professional medical advice, they can offer a snapshot of your gut microbiome's composition.
- Gut Microbiome Testing: More comprehensive than fundamental stool analysis, gut microbiome testing delves into the intricacies of your gut's bacterial ecosystem. These tests can reveal the richness and diversity of your microbiota, offering a benchmark against which you can measure the impact of dietary changes, probiotics, and lifestyle adjustments.

Using these tools, you can better understand your gut health's starting point and track changes over time, providing a data-driven approach to understanding improvements.

Quality of Life Indicators

While numbers and data provide one perspective, the qualitative changes in your day-to-day life are equally telling. Signs that your gut health is on the upswing can include:

- Elevated Energy Levels: A well-balanced gut can lead to more efficient digestion and nutrient absorption, boosting energy. If you find yourself less reliant on that mid-afternoon caffeine kick, it might be a sign of improved gut health.
- Enhanced Mood: A happier gut can contribute to a lighter mood thanks to the gut-brain axis. Notice if you experience fewer mood swings or a general uplift in your spirits.
- Reduced Digestive Discomfort: Perhaps the most obvious indicator is that a decrease in symptoms like bloating, gas, and irregular bowel movements signals that your gut health strategies are working.
- Better Sleep: As your gut health improves, you might find it easier to fall asleep and stay asleep, thanks to the balanced production of sleep-regulating neurotransmitters in the gut.

These quality-of-life improvements are tangible benefits reflecting the positive changes within your gut.

Long-Term Health Benefits

Beyond the immediate improvements, enhancing your gut health can have profound long-term effects on your overall health. Here are a few potential benefits to keep in mind:

- Strengthened Immune System: A robust gut microbiome supports the immune system. Over time, improved gut health can lead to fewer illnesses and a more resilient body.
- Lowered Risk of Chronic Diseases: Research suggests that a healthy gut can reduce the risk of developing chronic conditions such as obesity, type 2 diabetes, and heart disease. You're investing in your long-term wellness by supporting your gut health.
- Improved Mental Health: The ongoing dialogue between your gut and brain means that a healthy gut microbiome can reduce the risk of anxiety and depression.

Monitoring these long-term health markers, in conjunction with your healthcare provider, can further validate the effectiveness of your gut health regimen.

In sum, recognizing improvements in gut health involves a blend of self-observation, scientific tools, and an awareness of the broader impacts on your overall well-being. By paying attention to the whisper-quiet signs and the data-driven evidence, you can confidently and clearly navigate the path to optimal gut health.

9.5 COMBATING SKEPTICISM: WHY NATURAL REMEDIES DESERVE A PLACE IN YOUR GUT HEALTH TOOLKIT

In a world brimming with medical advancements and scientific breakthroughs, the whispers of nature's own medicine often go unheard. The skepticism surrounding natural remedies is as old as time. Yet, amidst the noise, a growing body of evidence suggests these age-old practices have more to offer than meets the eye, especially when nurturing our gut health. This isn't about dismissing modern medicine but rather about weaving the wisdom of natural remedies into the fabric of comprehensive gut care.

Natural remedies, from the humble ginger root to the probiotic-rich kefir, have danced through generations, offering gentle yet effective relief for many gut-related issues. However, the key to unlocking their potential lies not in blind faith but in approaching them with a discerning eye grounded in evidence-based practices.

Skepticism often stems from a need for more understanding or misconceptions about the efficacy and application of these remedies. At the intersection of tradition and science, integrative medicine offers a balanced perspective, harmonizing the best of both worlds for holistic gut health.

Integrative Medicine: Bridging the Gap

Integrative medicine emerges as a beacon of hope for those seeking a more rounded approach to gut health. This discipline does not simply stack natural remedies against conventional treatments but thoughtfully combines them, tailoring interventions to the individual's unique needs and health profile. The premise is simple yet profound: while traditional therapies target specific symptoms or diseases, natural remedies enhance the body's inherent healing mechanisms, often with fewer side effects.

Drawing on a wide array of practices, from herbal supplements to acupuncture, integrative medicine fosters a deeper understanding of health. It views the individual as a whole rather than a sum of disparate parts. This holistic lens focuses on gut health, acknowledging its pivotal role in our overall well-being and advocating for natural remedies as valuable tools in the gut health toolkit.

Research and Evidence: Sifting Through the Claims

As interest in natural remedies for gut health burgeons, so does the scrutiny of their claims. When considering any treatment option, it's crucial to differentiate between anecdotal evidence and scientific research. Several natural remedies have stood up to scientific rigor, demonstrating tangible benefits for gut health:

- Probiotic-rich foods like yogurt and kefir have shown promise in balancing gut microbiota, potentially easing conditions such as IBS.
- Prebiotic fibers in foods like garlic, onions, and bananas nourish beneficial gut bacteria, promoting a healthy digestive ecosystem.
- Herbal teas, such as peppermint and ginger, have been studied for their soothing effects on the gut, helping alleviate symptoms of indigestion and nausea.

This growing body of research lends credibility to specific natural remedies and paves the way for more informed choices in the quest for optimal gut health.

Personalized Approach: Tailoring Natural Remedies to Your Needs

The allure of natural remedies lies in their versatility and adaptability, catering to the unique tapestry of each individual's gut health. However, embracing these remedies necessitates a personalized approach that considers your specific health history, lifestyle, and existing conditions. Consulting with healthcare professionals familiar with conventional and natural treatments ensures a balanced strategy, marrying the strengths of each to your benefit.

- Assessment: A thorough evaluation of your gut health status, including ongoing treatments or medications, sets the stage for integrating natural remedies without adverse interactions.
- Customization: Tailoring remedies to address your unique challenges and goals enhances their effectiveness, ensuring they complement rather than complicate your health regimen.
- Monitoring: Tracking your response to natural remedies allows for adjustments as needed, optimizing outcomes and mitigating risks.

When thoughtfully integrated into your gut health strategy, natural remedies offer a bridge to a more harmonious state of well-being. Their potential to soothe, heal, and balance, supported by tradition and science, makes them an invaluable addition to our health arsenal.

As we wrap up this exploration into the realm of natural remedies and their place in gut health care, it's clear that skepticism, while healthy, should not deter us from considering all avenues of healing. The evidence supporting certain natural practices, coupled with an integrative approach and personalized strategies, underscores the potential of these time-honored remedies to enrich our journey toward better health. As we move forward, let us remain open to the possibilities of harnessing the best of both natural and conventional medicine for a holistic path to gut health and beyond.

CRAFTING YOUR PATH TO GUT HEALTH

Imagine you're planting a garden. You wouldn't just scatter seeds randomly and hope for the best. You'd start with a plan: assessing the soil, choosing the right plants, and setting achievable goals for your garden's growth. Similarly, improving your gut health starts with a clear, well-thought-out strategy. This chapter is about creating that plan, setting realistic goals, and making gradual changes that lead to lasting improvement in your gut health.

10.1 SETTING REALISTIC GOALS FOR GUT HEALTH IMPROVEMENT

SMART Goals

The first step is to set SMART goals: specific, measurable, achievable, relevant, and time-bound. It's like deciding precisely what you want your garden to look like by the end of the season. For gut health, a SMART goal might be, "I want to reduce my bloating by noting my food intake and symptoms daily for the next month to identify triggers." This goal is clear: you can measure progress by tracking your symptoms. It's undoubtedly achievable with commitment, directly related to improving gut health, and has a one-month deadline.

Baseline Assessment

Before you dive in, take a thorough inventory of your current gut health. This is akin to testing the soil and understanding what you're working with. Note your typical diet, any recurring symptoms (like bloating, gas, or irregular bowel movements), and how these symptoms impact your daily life. Tools like a food diary app or a simple notebook can be invaluable here.

Incremental Changes

Significant changes start with small steps. Instead of overhauling your diet overnight, focus on one change at a time. For example, if you're adding more fiber to your diet, include one extra serving of vegetables daily. This approach is similar to gradually adding plants rather than planting everything at once. It reduces feeling overwhelmed and makes it easier to stick with your plan.

Professional Consultation

Sometimes, you need more expertise. As you might consult a gardening expert to choose the best plants for your soil type, meeting with a healthcare professional can tailor your gut health goals to your needs, especially if you have existing health issues. A dietitian can provide personalized dietary advice, while a doctor can rule out more serious conditions that might be causing your symptoms.

Visual Element: An infographic including examples illustrating the steps to set SMART goals for gut health.

Textual Element: This is a checklist for conducting a baseline gut health assessment, with prompts for what to include in your food and symptom diary.

Improving your gut health isn't about quick fixes; it's about setting realistic goals, making small changes, and adjusting your plan as you learn more about what works for your body. With patience and persistence, you can create a thriving "garden" of gut health that supports your overall well-being.

10.2 TRACKING YOUR PROGRESS: TOOLS AND TECHNIQUES

Navigating the path to better gut health often feels like sailing through uncharted waters. To keep your ship steadily moving toward its destination, having a compass in the form of progress tracking is invaluable. This section will guide you through various methods to monitor your journey, offering clarity and insight into the effectiveness of your efforts.

Journaling

Introducing a daily journal as your companion on this voyage provides a space for reflection and observation. Here's how it works:

- Daily Entries: Each day, dedicate a few moments to jot down what you've eaten, any symptoms you've experienced, your mood, and overall well-being. It's akin to keeping a logbook on a ship, noting the conditions and events of the day.
- Patterns and Triggers: Over time, this logbook becomes a treasure trove of information, allowing you to spot patterns and identify triggers that affect your gut health. Certain foods consistently lead to discomfort, or stress is a significant factor.
- Adjustments: With this knowledge, you can tweak your diet and lifestyle. It's like adjusting your sails based on the wind direction, ensuring you're always moving forward, even if the route needs slight changes.

Digital Apps

In today's digital age, numerous apps are modern tools to track your progress. They offer features like:

- Food Tracking: Log your meals easily, often with nutritional breakdowns and the ability to scan barcodes for quick entry.
- Symptom Tracking: Some apps specialize in monitoring health symptoms, including those related to gut health, allowing you to note the severity and duration.
- Stool Quality: Yes, there are apps for this too! Monitoring stool quality can provide insights into your digestive health, indicating improvements or areas needing attention.

These digital companions can simplify the tracking process, making you more likely to stick with it. Plus, they often provide visual summaries of your data, helping you see your progress at a glance.

Although we can only suggest apps to you, here are our two favorites:

MyFitnessPal:

- Overview: Although primarily known as a calorie and exercise tracking app, MyFitnessPal can effectively monitor gut health. It allows users to track their food intake in detail, including macro- and micronutrients, which can help identify foods that benefit or harm gut health based on personal experience and symptoms.
- Features: It offers a comprehensive database of foods, including various brands and restaurant items, making it easier to log exactly what you're eating. You can also track your water intake, which is crucial for gut health, and customize your nutrition goals based on dietary advice or personal health objectives.

Cara Care:

- Overview: Cara Care is specifically designed to support individuals with digestive issues and is an excellent tool for those looking to improve their gut health. It offers personalized nutrition advice, symptom tracking, and the ability to connect with dietitians and medical professionals.

- Features: The app allows users to track their meals, symptoms, bowel movements, stress levels, and exercise, all of which can impact gut health. By analyzing this data, Cara Care can provide insights into how different aspects of lifestyle and diet correlate with gut health symptoms, helping users to make informed adjustments to their diet and lifestyle.

Both apps offer unique features that can assist in monitoring gut health and making necessary dietary and lifestyle adjustments. While MyFitnessPal provides a broad overview of dietary intake and its nutritional value, Cara Care offers a more targeted approach to managing digestive health and symptoms. Utilizing either of these apps can help individuals gain insights into their gut health and improve their overall well-being through personalized adjustments.

Biomarker Testing

For those who crave concrete data, periodic biomarker testing, such as microbiome analysis, offers a scientific method to assess changes in your gut health. These tests analyze your stool to evaluate the following:

- Microbial Diversity: A healthy gut hosts various bacteria. These tests can show increases in diversity, a sign of improved gut health.
- Beneficial vs. Harmful Bacteria: Get insights into the balance of beneficial versus harmful bacteria and how this balance shifts in response to your gut health efforts.
- Inflammation Markers: Some tests can identify markers

of inflammation in the gut, providing clues about underlying issues that may need addressing.

While these tests provide a snapshot of your gut's health at a given time, tracking changes through repeated testing can offer a clear picture of your progress over time.

Reflective Practice

Beyond the logs, apps, and tests, taking time for regular reflection is a powerful tool. Here's how you might approach this:

- Weekly Reflections: Each week, set aside time to review your journal entries and app data. Consider what went well, what challenges arose, and how you felt overall.
- Learnings: Identify critical learnings from the week. You may have discovered a new trigger food or found that meditation helped soothe your symptoms.
- Adjustments: Based on your reflections, plan any adjustments for the coming week. This might involve tweaking your diet, trying new stress-reduction techniques, or setting a goal to increase your physical activity.
- Motivation: Reflect on your motivation levels and what's driving you. Recognizing your motivation can help you stay the course, especially during challenging times.

This reflective practice turns your journey into a learning experience, where each step, whether forward or backward, provides valuable insights that shape your path to better gut health.

You create a detailed map of your journey by employing these tools and techniques to track your progress. This map helps you navigate the complex waters of gut health and empowers you to make informed decisions, adjust your course as needed, and ultimately, reach your destination of improved well-being.

10.3 ADJUSTING YOUR PLAN: WHEN TO PIVOT AND WHY

Navigating the world of gut health is akin to tending a garden through the changing seasons. Just as a gardener listens to the weather and adapts their planting, watering, and harvesting strategies, so must we attune ourselves to our body's signals and be prepared to modify our gut health regimen as needed. This adaptability is not a sign of setback but rather an intelligent response to the evolving landscape of our body's needs.

Listening to Your Body

The cornerstone of any effective gut health plan is listening and responding to your body's feedback. Your body communicates in various ways, from the subtle whisper of mild discomfort to the loud protest of a painful symptom. The art lies in tuning into these signals without immediate judgment or dismissal, allowing them to guide your decisions. For instance, if a food that once seemed beneficial now consistently leads to discomfort, it might be time to reconsider its place in your diet. Similarly, a new lifestyle habit that was meant to reduce stress but instead adds to it may need reevaluation.

Signs You Need to Adjust

Recognizing when to adjust your gut health plan is crucial. Here are some indicators that it might be time for a change:

- Persistent Symptoms: If symptoms like bloating, gas, or irregular bowel movements continue despite your efforts, this is a clear sign that your current approach needs tweaking.
- New Health Issues: The emergence of new symptoms or health concerns can indicate that your body's needs have changed, necessitating a shift in your gut health strategy.
- Lack of Progress: If you need to see improvements or achieve the milestones you set, consider alternative approaches.
- Increased Stress or Discomfort: If any part of your gut health regimen is causing more stress or discomfort rather than alleviating it, this is a sign that adjustments are needed.

Seeking Expert Advice

At particular crossroads, professional guidance can illuminate the path forward. Whether it's a persistent symptom that defies explanation or the consideration of a new supplement or dietary change, consulting with a healthcare professional ensures that your adjustments are informed and safe. A dietitian can offer nuanced advice on food choices, while a doctor might identify underlying conditions that require specific interventions. Think of these professionals as your co-navigators, offering their expertise to help steer your plan in the right direction.

Iterative Process

Understanding that pursuing optimal gut health is an iterative process can transform how you approach adjustments. Each step, whether forward or sideways, is part of a more extensive process of learning and growth. This perspective encourages a proactive, rather than reactive, stance towards changes. It invites experimentation, where trying a new probiotic, eliminating a suspected trigger food, or incorporating a stress-reduction practice is seen as gathering data rather than a make-or-break decision.

This approach also fosters resilience. When a strategy doesn't yield the expected results, instead of viewing it as a failure, it's seen as valuable feedback informing your next steps. It's a cycle of observing, adjusting, and observing again, much like a scientist in a lab, where each iteration brings you closer to understanding your body's unique language and needs.

In practice, this might look like:

- Trial Periods for New Changes: Introduce one change at a time and give it a trial period. Monitor your body's response and decide whether to continue, adjust, or discontinue based on the outcomes.
- Regular Check-ins: Schedule regular intervals, perhaps monthly or quarterly, to review your gut health plan. Assess what's working, what's not, and what might need to change.
- Openness to New Information: Stay informed about the latest research and developments in gut health. New findings might prompt adjustments to your plan.

- Feedback Loops: Create a feedback loop where you regularly consult with healthcare professionals, revisit your goals and progress, and adjust your plan based on the accumulated insights.

By embracing the iterative nature of this process, you are equipped to navigate the dynamic landscape of gut health with agility and confidence. Adjustments become necessary and welcomed steps on the path to understanding and nurturing your body's intricate ecosystem. This adaptive journey, marked by attentive listening, informed decision-making, and continual learning, lays the groundwork for lasting improvements in gut health and, by extension, your overall quality of life.

10.4 COMMUNITY SUPPORT: FINDING YOUR GUT HEALTH TRIBE

The path to optimal gut health can sometimes feel like a solitary climb up a steep hill. However, the journey becomes a shared adventure when you find a group of fellow climbers, each with their own insights and experiences. This section unveils the significance of community in gut health, guiding you on connecting with or even creating a network of support that enriches your quest for wellness.

The Power of Shared Experiences

A supportive community offers more than camaraderie; it is a vital resource for knowledge, encouragement, and empathy. When you share your experiences, you're likely to discover others who have faced similar challenges and can offer practical advice or simply a listening ear. This exchange fosters a sense of belonging and can significantly lighten the mental and emotional load often accompanying health issues.

Navigating Online Forums and Social Media

In the digital age, online platforms have become bustling hubs where people from all corners of the globe connect over common interests, including gut health. Here's how to tap into these virtual communities:

- Research: Look for forums and social media groups dedicated to gut health, digestive disorders, or general wellness. Websites like Reddit and platforms like Facebook host numerous groups where members share advice, success stories, and support.
- Engagement: Once you've found a community that resonates with you, dive in. Introduce yourself, share your story, and participate in discussions. Remember, the more you engage, the more you stand to gain from the collective wisdom of the group.
- Discernment: While these communities are invaluable, it's crucial to approach the information shared with discernment. Not all advice will be applicable or beneficial to your unique situation. When in doubt, consult a healthcare professional to corroborate any advice you're considering.

Seeking Out Local Support Groups

While online communities offer convenience and a broad reach, local support groups provide a tangible connection that only face-to-face interaction can. Here's how to find these groups:

- Local Health Clinics and Hospitals: Many health institutions run support groups for individuals dealing with various health issues, including those related to gut health. Contact clinics and hospitals in your area to inquire about such groups.
- Community Centers and Libraries: These local hubs often host workshops, talks, and groups on various topics, including nutrition and wellness. Check their event calendars for upcoming gut health-related activities.
- Yoga Studios and Wellness Centers: Places focused on overall well-being sometimes offer sessions or groups centered around holistic health practices, including diet and gut health. These settings can provide a serene backdrop for learning and sharing.

Creating Your Support System

If your search for the perfect support group is empty, why not start your own? Here's a blueprint for creating a community:

- Define Your Vision: What do you hope to achieve with this group? Whether it's sharing recipes and tips or simply offering support, having a clear purpose will help attract like-minded individuals.
- Utilize Social Media: Platforms like Facebook and Meetup simplify creating and promoting groups. Use these tools to organize your group, schedule meetings, and share information.
- Partner with Local Businesses: Contact health food stores, wellness centers, and yoga studios to see if they would be interested in hosting or promoting your group. They might also provide expert speakers for your meetings.

- Set a Regular Schedule: Whether it's a weekly coffee meet-up or a monthly workshop, having a regular schedule makes it easier for people to commit and participate actively.

Visual Element: This is a step-by-step infographic on starting your gut health support group, covering everything from defining your vision to promoting your meetings.

Textual Element: A "How to Connect" guide offering tips for engaging with online communities, approaching local institutions for support group information, and leveraging social media to grow your group.

In essence, finding or creating a tribe of individuals who understand the ups and downs of gut health can transform your journey from a solitary venture into a shared exploration. This tribe becomes a source of motivation, inspiration, and collective wisdom, empowering you to navigate the complexities of gut health with confidence and support.

10.5 STAYING MOTIVATED: CELEBRATING WINS AND OVERCOMING SETBACKS

Achieving optimal gut health is a process filled with highs and lows, like navigating through a dense forest. In moments of progress, the path is clear, and the journey feels rewarding. Yet, when faced with challenges, the way forward can seem obscured. It's during these times that maintaining motivation becomes crucial. Here's how to keep the momentum, celebrate your progress, and gracefully move through the inevitable setbacks.

Recognizing Small Wins

Every step toward better gut health, no matter how minor it might seem, is a victory worth celebrating. These moments of progress are the beacons of light guiding you through the forest, reminding you that you're on the right path. Whether it's a day without discomfort, trying a new gut-friendly recipe, or simply remembering to take your probiotic, acknowledging these wins can uplift your spirits and reinforce your commitment to your health. Make it a habit to reflect on these positive moments by noting them in your journal or sharing them with your support group. This practice boosts your morale and helps build a mindset focused on growth and gratitude.

Dealing with Setbacks

Setbacks are natural occurrences on the road to better health. They're not roadblocks but detours that offer learning and adaptation opportunities. When faced with a setback, consider the following strategies:

- Reframe the Experience: Instead of seeing it as a failure, view it as valuable feedback. What can this setback teach you about your body's needs or how you can fine-tune your approach?
- Adjust Your Plan: Use this feedback to make informed adjustments to your gut health regimen. A particular food doesn't agree with you as you thought, or you need to incorporate more stress-reduction practices into your routine.

- Seek Support: Turn to your support community for advice and encouragement. Often, others have been through similar experiences and can offer insights or simply lend a sympathetic ear.

Maintaining a Long-Term Perspective

Improving gut health is a long-term endeavor. It's helpful to zoom out and view your efforts from a broader perspective, acknowledging that progress takes time. This wider lens allows you to see beyond the immediate obstacles and recognize the overall upward trend in your health journey. Patience is key. Trust that the small, consistent actions you're taking now will accumulate and lead to significant improvements over time.

Self-Compassion and Patience

The most critical component of staying motivated is practicing self-compassion. Be kind to yourself, especially during moments of frustration or when progress seems slow. Remember, you're doing your best, and your efforts are valid and valuable. Allow yourself the grace to move at your own pace, understanding that each body is unique and responds differently to changes in diet and lifestyle. Patience and self-compassion lay the foundation for a sustainable and fulfilling journey toward better gut health.

In closing, remember that the path to improved gut health, much like any significant life change, is marked by a series of steps and adjustments. Celebrating the small wins lights the way forward while learning from setbacks enriches your understanding and resilience. Keeping a long-term perspective and practicing self-compassion ensure that you navigate this path with patience and kindness toward yourself. As we move into the next chapter, we'll build on these principles, exploring further strategies to enhance your gut health and, consequently, your overall quality of life.

KEEPING THE GAME ALIVE

Now that you've unlocked the secrets to transformative gut health, it's time to share your newfound wisdom and guide others to the same path of wellness.

By sharing your honest thoughts about "Gut Health Unlocked" on Amazon, you become a beacon for fellow seekers of better health. Your review doesn't just reflect your journey; it illuminates the way for others who are still searching for answers to their gut health puzzles.

Thank you sincerely for your support. The journey to better gut health thrives on shared knowledge, and with your help, we're extending a helping hand to many more individuals eager to improve their lives.

The message of gut health continues to spread far and wide thanks to champions like you. Together, we're not just reading about change; we're leading it.

Scan the QR code to leave your review on Amazon.

Your contribution is more than just a review; it's a vital part of keeping the gut health revolution going. Thank you for being an invaluable member of our community and for helping us to pass on the torch of health and well-being.

CONCLUSION

As we reach the closing pages of our journey together, I'm grateful for the steps we've embarked on toward unlocking the mysteries of gut health, especially for those of us navigating the complexities of life over 40. From the foundational understanding of our gut's ecosystem to the nuanced strategies of diet, lifestyle adjustments, and overcoming the hurdles that often stand in our way, we've traversed a path that underscores a holistic approach to nurturing our digestive well-being.

I aim to illuminate the truth that there's no universal solution to gut health. The uniqueness of our bodies, lifestyles, and needs demands a personalized approach. This book has sought to equip you with the tools to tailor your diet, recalibrate your lifestyle, and manage stress in ways that resonate with your circumstances. Remember, the dietary strategies and lifestyle changes we've explored are not prescriptions but invitations to experiment and find what indeed works for you.

We've delved into the interconnectedness of gut health, not just as a cornerstone of digestive wellness but as a pivotal force in our overall health landscape. The gut-brain axis, the microbiome's extensive role in our bodily functions, from mood regulation to immune defense, underscores the profound impact that nurturing gut health can have on our lives. This is a testament to the idea that caring for our gut is, in essence, caring for our whole self.

In our shared quest for gut health, key strategies have emerged as beacons: embracing a diverse and nutrient-rich diet; making stress reduction and quality sleep non-negotiable; engaging in regular, gentle exercise; and not underestimating the power of staying hydrated and sticking to a nurturing routine. These pillars form the foundation of a gut-friendly lifestyle that can steer us towards better digestion and enhanced vitality.

I invite you to take the first or next step on your gut health journey. Apply the insights and advice that resonate with you, experiment with mindful adjustments, and don't hesitate to seek guidance from healthcare professionals to navigate this path confidently.

But remember, the journey to optimal gut health is perpetual, evolving with each new piece of research, with every shift in our bodies, and with time. Stay curious, be open to adapting your approach, and listen intently to the signals your body sends you.

I encourage you to share your stories of triumphs and trials in improving gut health. Whether through social media, in conversations with loved ones, or within community groups, your story can inspire and uplift others embarking on similar journeys. There's immense power in our shared experiences, fostering a community of support and understanding that can make the journey less daunting.

As an added bonus, here is a link to a site which provides many of the supplements that were alluded to in this book. Please take a look as you venture into your gut health journey.

https://us.fullscript.com/welcome/healthy-solutions-md

In closing, let me affirm your capability to positively influence your gut health and, by extension, your overall well-being. No matter where you're starting from, the steps you take towards nurturing your gut are steps towards a more vibrant, healthful life. It's always possible to make changes that bring about profound benefits. Here's to your health, happiness, and a well-traveled journey of discovery and renewal.

With heartfelt wishes for your continued health and well-being,

Denise Smith Marsh

REFERENCES

- *The gut-brain axis: interactions between enteric microbiota, ...* https://www.ncbi.nlm.nih.gov/pmc/articles/PMC4367209/
- *The Human Microbiome and Its Impacts on Health - PMC - NCBI* https://www.ncbi.nlm.nih.gov/pmc/articles/PMC7306068/
- *Digestion in the Stomach - Food Enzyme Institute* https://www.foodenzymeinstitute.com/content/Digestion-in-the-Stomach.aspx
- *Leaky Gut and the Ingredients That Help Treat It: A Review* https://www.ncbi.nlm.nih.gov/pmc/articles/PMC9862683/
- *Probiotics Regulate Gut Microbiota: An Effective Method to ...* https://www.ncbi.nlm.nih.gov/pmc/articles/PMC8512487/
- *Prevalence of non-celiac gluten sensitivity - Dr. Schär Institute* https://www.drschaer.com/us/institute/a/non-celiac-gluten-sensitivity-epidemiology#:
- *Detox diets for toxin elimination and weight management* https://pubmed.ncbi.nlm.nih.gov/25522674/
- *Controversies and Recent Developments of the Low- ...* https://www.ncbi.nlm.nih.gov/pmc/articles/PMC5390324/
- *Foods that fight inflammation - Harvard Health* https://www.health.harvard.edu/staying-healthy/foods-that-fight-inflammation
- *Could fish oil fight inflammation? - American Heart Association* https://www.heart.org/en/news/2019/12/12/could-fish-oil-fight-inflammation
- *How To Pick the Best Probiotic* https://health.clevelandclinic.org/how-to-pick-the-best-probiotic-for-you
- *Fermented Foods: 50+ Recipes to Get You Started* https://www.attainable-sustainable.net/ferment-vegetables/
- *Non-Celiac Gluten Sensitivity | BeyondCeliac.org* https://www.beyondceliac.org/celiac-disease/non-celiac-gluten-sensitivity/
- *The 3 phases of the low FODMAP diet* https://www.monashfodmap.com/blog/3-phases-low-fodmap-diet/
- *The ketogenic diet: its impact on human gut microbiota and ...* https://www.ncbi.nlm.nih.gov/pmc/articles/PMC9876773/
- *Nutritional Status and the Influence of the Vegan Diet on ...* https://www.ncbi.nlm.nih.gov/pmc/articles/PMC7073751/

REFERENCES

- *Stress & the gut-brain axis: Regulation by the microbiome* https://www.ncbi.nlm.nih.gov/pmc/articles/PMC5736941/
- *Mindful Eating: A Review Of How The Stress-Digestion ...* https://www.ncbi.nlm.nih.gov/pmc/articles/PMC7219460/
- *How Gut Health Impacts Sleep (And Vice Versa)* https://www.sleep.com/sleep-health/how-gut-health-impacts-sleep
- *Exercise Modifies the Gut Microbiota with Positive Health ...* https://www.ncbi.nlm.nih.gov/pmc/articles/PMC5357536/
- *Water, Hydration and Health - PMC* https://www.ncbi.nlm.nih.gov/pmc/articles/PMC2908954/
- *Interactions Between Gut Microbiota, Host, and Herbal ...* https://www.ncbi.nlm.nih.gov/pmc/articles/PMC7379170/
- *A gastroenterologist's morning routine* https://www.fdhs.com/morning-routine-of-a-gut-health-doc/#:
- *Improve Your Gut-Brain Connection (and Your Mood) In 3 ...* https://www.mindful.org/3-ways-to-improve-your-gut-brain-connection-and-your-mood/
- *Abdominal Bloating: Causes, Remedies, and More* https://www.healthline.com/health/abdominal-bloating
- *Dietary Fiber for Constipation: How Much You Need* https://www.webmd.com/digestive-disorders/dietary-fiber-the-natural-solution-for-constipation
- *Probiotics for Diarrhea: Types, Uses, Side Effects, Benefits* https://www.webmd.com/digestive-disorders/probiotics-diarrhea
- *How to Do an Elimination Diet and Why - Healthline* https://www.healthline.com/nutrition/elimination-diet
- *Strain-specific impacts of probiotics are a significant driver ...* https://www.nature.com/articles/s41564-022-01213-w
- *The Gut-Brain Axis: Influence of Microbiota on Mood and ...* https://www.ncbi.nlm.nih.gov/pmc/articles/PMC6469458/
- *Is the secret to successful aging in your gut?* https://www.womenshealthmag.com/uk/food/a45651063/gut-health-and-ageing/
- *10 research-backed ways to improve gut health* https://www.medicalnewstoday.com/articles/325293
- *Using the SMART-EST Goals in Lifestyle Medicine Prescription* https://www.ncbi.nlm.nih.gov/pmc/articles/PMC7232896/#:
- *5 Powerful Health Benefits of Journaling* https://intermountainhealthcare.org/blogs/5-powerful-health-benefits-of-journaling
- *Microbiome tests: What to know - Medical News Today* https://www.medicalnewstoday.com/articles/microbiome-testing#:

- *Support Groups: Getting the Help You Need* https://iffgd.org/support-groups-getting-the-help-you-need/
- Lamba, P., Sharma, D., & Sinnarkar, V. (2022). *Polycystic Ovarian Syndrome Treated with Individualized Homeopathy: A Case Report.* Alternative Therapies in Health and Medicine, 28(6), 60-64.
- Nucci, D., Nardi, M., Provenzano, S., Gianfredi, V., & Gianfredi, V. (2021). *Wikipedia, Google Trends and Diet: Assessment of Temporal Trends in the Internet Users' Searches in Italy before and during COVID-19 Pandemic.* Nutrients, 13(11), 3683.
- Gianfredi, V., Nucci, D., Nucci, D., Nardi, M., & Provenzano, S. (2023). *Using Google Trends and Wikipedia to Investigate the Global Public's Interest in the Pancreatic Cancer Diagnosis of a Celebrity.* International Journal of Environmental Research and Public Health, 20(3), 2106.
- Tchounwou, P., & Han, O. (2013). *International Journal of Environmental Research and Public Health Best Paper Award 2013.* International Journal of Environmental Research and Public Health, 10(1), 443-5.

Printed in Great Britain
by Amazon